Leicestershire Partners

NHS Trust

The Frith Prescribing Guidelines
for Adults with Learning Disability

Prescribing Guidelines for Adults with Learning Disability

Leicestershire Partnership **NHS**

NHS Trust

Sabyasachi Bhaumik
David Branford

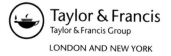
Taylor & Francis
Taylor & Francis Group

LONDON AND NEW YORK

© 2005 Leicestershire Partnership NHS Trust

First published in 2005 by Taylor & Francis, an imprint of the Taylor & Francis Group, 2 Park Square, Milton Park, Abingdon, Oxfordshire, OX14 4RN

Tel.:   +44 (0) 20 7017 6000
Fax.:   +44 (0) 20 7017 6699
E-mail: info.medicine@tandf.co.uk
Website: http://www.tandf.co.uk/medicine

Although every effort has been made to ensure that all owners of copyright material have been acknowledged in this publication, we would be glad to acknowledge in subsequent reprints or editions any omissions brought to our attention.

Although every effort has been made to ensure that drug doses and other information are presented accurately in this publication, the ultimate responsibility rests with the prescribing physician. Neither the publishers nor the authors can be held responsible for errors or for any consequences arising from the use of information contained herein. For detailed prescribing information or instructions on the use of any product or procedure discussed herein, please consult the prescribing information or instructional material issued by the manufacturer.

A CIP record for this book is available from the British Library.

ISBN 1–84184–573–6

Distributed in the USA by
Fulfilment Center
Taylor & Francis
10650 Tobben Drive
Independence, KY 41051, USA
Toll Free Tel.: +1 800 634 7064
E-mail: taylorandfrancis@thomsonlearning.com

Distributed in Canada by
Taylor & Francis
74 Rolark Drive
Scarborough, Ontario M1R 4G2, Canada
Toll Free Tel.: +1 877 226 2237
E-mail: tal_fran@istar.ca

Distributed in the rest of the world by
Thomson Publishing Services
Cheriton House
North Way
Andover, Hampshire SP10 5BE, UK
Tel.: +44 (0)1264 332424
E-mail: salesorder.tandf@thomsonpublishingservices.co.uk

Composition by J&L Composition, Filey, North Yorkshire

Printed and bound by Cromwell Press Ltd, Trowbridge, Wiltshire

Contents

Authors and editors

Editors: Dr S Bhaumik
                          Dr D Branford

Assistant Editor: Dr D M Michael

Authors: Dr S Bhaumik
                          Dr S Nadkarni
                          Dr J M Watson
                          Dr L B Raju
                          Dr A Biswas
                          Dr R T Alexander
                          Dr D M Michael
                          Dr K Bretherton
                          Dr S K Gangadharan

Preface

This is the first attempt to produce prescribing guidelines for adults with learning disability especially in relation to the management of epilepsy, behaviour disorders and functional psychiatric illnesses. The diagnosis of psychiatric disorders in this population is fraught with difficulties due to lack of standardized diagnostic criteria, significant communication difficulties and co-morbidities such as epilepsy and physical health problems. Clinicians working in this speciality tend to depend on the evidence from mainstream psychiatry and the experience shared with other colleagues, due to a scarcity of reliable evidence of drug treatment. Though all people with learning disability share certain features of delayed development, they are a heterogeneous group, and therefore their clinical presentation and response to treatment may vary considerably. In many instances psychiatrists may have to rely on direct observation and information gathered from carers. This applies not only in arriving at a diagnostic formulation but also in monitoring the outcome of treatment including any adverse events.

These guidelines are a result of influences drawn from the existing evidence base and from the consensus opinion of a number of experienced clinicians. Without the input from these colleagues, this book would not serve its purpose.

Sabyasachi Bhaumik
29 October 2004

Contributors

Dr R Alexander
Dr T Betts
Dr S Bhaumik
Dr A B Biswas
Dr K Bretherton
Professor S Deb
Dr S K Gangadharan
Dr D M Michael
Dr S Nadkarni
Dr L B Raju
Dr J M Watson

Acknowledgements

I particularly wish to thank my retired colleague Dr Agnes Hauck, who has been a source of inspiration to all of us in working towards developing these guidelines.

Dr D Bagalkote
Dr M Bambrick
Dr M Barrett
Dr E Beber
Dr E Bonell
Dr P Bown
Dr D Chavda
Dr M Churchard
Dr P Cutajar
Dr A Dasgupta
Ms R Davda
Dr J Devapriam
Dr S Elcock
Dr E M R de Saram
Dr C de Souza
Ms T Finamore
Dr I J Gunaratne
Dr A Hauck
Ms L Hayes
Ms W Hickling
Ms C C Hill
Dr S Hoare
Dr B Houghton
Dr A Imre
Dr A R Khan
Dr Jaydeokar
Dr S Johnston
Dr J Jones
Dr P Karri

Dr R Lansdall-Welfare
Ms S Lyons
Ms V MacDonald
Dr F McKenzie
Ms L McManus
Dr R Madina
Dr S Majumdar
Dr T Marshall
Ms J May
Dr I Mitra
Ms M Mitchell
Ms L Moore
Dr T Mukherjee
Dr C L Narayana
Dr M Nath
Dr B Nwulu
Ms L O'Neill
Ms C Plumb
Dr V Ram
Dr S Rao
Dr O H Rauf
Dr J Roberts
Dr K M Sidahmed
Dr P Speight
Dr M Tajuddin
Dr N Taylor
Dr N Tin
Dr D N Wilson

Abbreviations

5-HT	5-hydroxytryptamine	LD	learning disability
AAMR	American Association of Mental Retardation	MAOI	monoamine oxidase inhibitor
		MRI	magnetic resonance imaging
ABC	aberrent behaviour checklist	NADPH	nicotinamide adenine dinucleotide phosphate reduced form
ABS	adaptive behaviour scale		
ADHD	attention deficit hyperactivity disorder		
		NARI	noradrenaline re-uptake inhibitors
AED	antiepileptic drugs		
AIMS	abnormal involuntary movement scale	NASSA	noradrenergic and specific serotonergic antidepressant
APP	amyloid precursor protein	NICE	National Institute for Clinical Excellence
ASD	autistic spectrum disorder		
BNF	British National Formulary	NMDA	N-methyl-D-aspartate
CB	challenging behaviour	OCD	obsessive compulsive disorder
CSM	Committee on the Safety of Medicines	PDD	pervasive developmental disorder
CT	computerised tomography	PET	positron emission tomography
CYP	cytochrome P450		
DASH	Diagnostic Assessment for the Severely Handicapped	PIMRA	Psychopathology Inventory for Mentally Retarded Adults
DC-LD	Diagnostic Criteria for psychiatric disorders for use with adults with Learning Disabilities/mental retardation	PKU	phenylketonuria
		PR	per rectum
		QTc	corrected QT interval in the ECG
		RSS	relatives stress scale
DMR	Dementia questionnaire for Mentally Retarded persons	SCAN	schedules of clinical assessment and neuropsychiatry
DSM-IV	Diagnostic and Statistical Manual of mental disorders, 1994	SIB	self injurious behaviour
		SJW	St John's wort
ECG	electrocardiography	SNRI	serotonin noradrenaline re-uptake inhibitors
ECT	electroconvulsive therapy		
EEG	electroencephalogram	SOD	superoxide dismutase
FMR	fragile X mental retardation	SPECT	single photon emission computerized tomography.
GABA	γ-amino butyric acid		
HD	hyperactivity disorder	SSRI	selective serotonin re-uptake inhibitors
ICD-10	International Classification of Disorders		
		SXR	steroid and xenobiotic receptors
IM	intramuscular		
IQ	intelligence quotient	T3	thyronine
IV	intravenous	TCA	tricyclic antidepressants

Learning disability

Definition

There is a general consensus on the concept of **learning disability** (LD). It requires the presence of three criteria based on the definition derived after extensive consultation in the USA (American Association on Mental Retardation, 1992):

Definition of learning disability

- a significant developmental intellectual impairment *and*
- concurrent deficits in social functioning or adaptive behaviour *and*
- the condition is manifest before the age of 18 years.

Significant intellectual impairment is usually defined as an intelligence quotient (IQ) more than two standard deviations below the general population mean (originally fixed at 100). This is an IQ below 70 on recognized IQ tests. 2% of the population have an IQ below this level.

Significant deficits in social functioning are commonly measured by the Vineland Adaptive Behaviour Scales. These assess communication, daily living skills, socialization and motor skills.

People with LD have significantly more health problems than the rest of the population. Around 50% have a major psychiatric or behaviour problem requiring specialist help, 25% have active epilepsy and at least 33% have a sensory impairment. Around 40% have associated major physical disabilities of mobility and incontinence. These substantial health needs are often overlooked or unmet. Moreover, 50–90% of people with LD have communication difficulties; and a lack of supported communication may compound their problems in receiving the health care that they need.

The term **learning difficulty**, first proposed by the Warnock Committee, is a much broader category than LD. This is the term used in the UK education system. Learning difficulty includes speech and language impairments; learning problems arising from sensory impairments, physical disabilities, medical problems or behaviour difficulties; and specific learning problems such as dyslexia. LD is associated with global impairment of intellectual and adaptive functioning and is assessed by *intellectual* criteria. Learning difficulty is assessed by *educational* criteria. The measures for the latter are mostly proxy measures of learning achievement (rather than the learning process itself) such as memory recall, reading, number and problem solving. It is estimated that about one in five children has a learning difficulty at some time during the course of life. One in six children has a learning difficulty at any one time. These guidelines refer to adults with LD, and learning difficulties will not be considered further.

Prevalence

The prevalence of LD depends on the cut-off point used for the definition of LD (Table 1.1) and the methodology used to measure it. Studies that have screened whole populations tend to find a higher prevalence (around 6 per 1000 population) than those that include only those known to services, the administrative prevalence. It is estimated that the prevalence is increasing at the rate of 1% a year.

Table 1.1 Administrative prevalence of LD in the UK		
Severity of LD	*IQ*	*Prevalence per 1000 population*
Mild	50–69	30
Moderate	35–49	3
Severe	20–34	
Profound	<20	0.5

Aetiology

Biological, environmental and social factors may contribute to the development of LD. A large number of different aetiological processes may be involved; these are usually complex and often not completely understood. Biological factors are present in about 67–75% of people with LD, the majority operating before birth (Table 1.2). The two most common genetic causes are Down syndrome and fragile X syndrome. In a third of people with LD, no primary diagnosis can be made.

Table 1.2 Biological factors that may cause LD

Period of origin	Nature of disorder	Common examples
Prenatal period	**Genetic disorders**	
	Chromosome aberrations	Down syndrome (trisomy 21)
	Single gene mutations	Tuberous sclerosis, phenylketonuria, mucopolysaccharidoses, fragile X syndrome
	Microdeletions	Prader–Willi syndrome, Williams syndrome
	Congenital malformations	
	Central nervous system malformations	Neural tube defects
	Multiple malformation syndromes	Cornelia de Lange syndrome
	Exposure	
	Maternal infections	Congenital rubella, HIV
	Teratogens	Foetal alcohol syndrome
	Toxaemia, placental insufficiency	Prematurity
	Severe malnutrition	Intrauterine growth retardation
	Trauma	Physical injury
	Iatrogenic	Radiation, drugs
Perinatal period	Infections	TORCH infections: toxoplasmosis, hepatitis B, syphilis, herpes zoster, rubella, cytomegalovirus, herpes simplex
	Delivery	Anoxic brain damage
	Other causes	Hyperbilirubinaemia
Postnatal period	Infections	Encephalitis
	Metabolic	Hypoglycaemia
	Endocrine	Hypothyroidism (cretinism)
	Cerebrovascular	Thromboembolic phenomena
	Toxins	Lead poisoning
	Trauma	Head injury
	Neoplasms	Meningioma, craniopharyngioma
	Psychosocial factors	Understimulation
Any	Untraceable or unknown	

Key points specific to learning disability

Communication

Difficulties in communication may make it more difficult for the doctor to ascertain the nature and extent of any benefits and the side effects of prescribing a drug for a patient with LD. When a patient is living independently, it is crucial to communicate the need to take the medicine and the instructions for taking it. Simple written or pictorial instructions may help understanding and compliance. It may be prudent to ensure that support is in place to monitor that the drug is taken and, if required, to monitor blood levels of the drug. When a patient is being cared for by others, it is important that the carers understand the purpose of the medicine, how it should be given and what parameters need to be monitored. When eliciting and giving information about epilepsy and other complex phenomena, clear simple language should be used rather than medical terms.

Consent

Whenever possible, express consent should be obtained from the patient before beginning treatment. This is in accordance with General Medical Council guidance. Express consent usually means consent that is expressed orally or in writing. However, where an individual cannot speak or write, other forms of communication may be sufficient.

For an individual's consent to be legally valid and professionally acceptable, the individual must be capable of taking that particular decision (competent), be acting voluntarily and be provided with enough information (in a form that he can understand) to enable him to make the decision. For adults with LD, this is often a process rather than a one-off effort. Legally, capacity to give consent is assumed until the contrary is shown.

Broadly, incapacity means that an individual is unable by reason of mental disability to make a decision for himself on the matter in question or is unable to communicate that decision. No one can give consent for an incompetent adult.

The assessment of an adult patient's capacity to make a decision about his own medical treatment is a matter for clinical judgement guided by professional practice and is subject to legal requirements. It is the personal responsibility of any doctor proposing to treat a patient to judge whether the patient has the capacity to give valid consent. The doctor has a duty to give the patient an account in simple terms of the benefits and risks of the proposed treatment and to explain the other principal options.

Demonstrating an individual's capacity

An individual should be able to:

- understand in simple language what the medical treatment is, its purpose and nature, and why it is being proposed
- understand its principal benefits, risks and other options
- understand in broad terms what will be the consequences of *not* receiving the proposed treatment
- retain the information for long enough to make an effective decision
- weigh that information in the balance and arrive at a free choice.

NB: All assessments of a patient's capacity should be fully recorded in the patient's medical notes.

However, there are occasions when some forms of medical treatment are lawful in the absence of the patient's consent. The **concept of necessity** permits doctors to provide treatment without obtaining consent if:

- there is a **necessity to act** when it is not practicable to communicate with the assisted person *and*
- the action taken is such that a reasonable person would take, given all the circumstances, acting in the **best interests** of the assisted person.

Not only may a doctor give treatment to an incapacitated patient when it is clearly in that person's best interests but it is also a common law duty to do so.

For most low-level decisions, there should generally be agreement between health professionals, the incapacitated person in so far as he can express a view and people close to him. Parents, carers and other people close to the patient may be able to provide information about his preferences, needs and best interests. Simple diagnostic or treatment options, such as taking blood samples for anaemia or lithium levels or prescribing an antibiotic for an infection or a mild analgesic for a headache, are uncontroversial. Treatment decisions that are so serious that they require a court decision are beyond the scope of these guidelines.

The principles and procedures for the detention of an individual for assessment or treatment or other purposes under the provisions of the Mental Health Act 1983 are the same as for the general population. Further details are beyond the scope of these guidelines.

Need for guidelines

About 50% of adults with LD have a psychiatric or behaviour problem; and 25% have active epilepsy. In this population, both the diagnosis and treatment of these common problems may need a different approach from that in the general population. Although there are guidelines to assist practitioners in prescribing drugs for mental health problems in the wider population, these are the first guidelines to address the specific issues relating to the pharmacological treatment of mental health problems in adults with LD.

Psychiatric and behaviour problems often present differently in adults with LD from the ways in which they do in the general population. In addition, symptoms of an underlying physical condition or a reaction to environmental changes may mask those of an additional psychiatric disturbance. Difficulties in diagnosis may be further compounded by the communication difficulties experienced by people with LD. For many conditions, there is a lack of suitable diagnostic criteria or instruments.

In the psychiatry of LD, the evidence base for the use of psychotropic drugs is extremely limited. There are few well-designed randomized, controlled trials. Adults with LD frequently have additional health problems that preclude them from being recruited into studies. The National Institute for Clinical Excellence (NICE) has not yet produced guidelines specifically for the LD population. Consequently, a wide range of psychotropic drugs are used outside their licensed indications to manage challenging behaviours, which may or may not be associated with an underlying mental health problem. For example, 23% of the LD population are prescribed antipsychotics for behavioural disturbances. The reasons for this include pressure from professionals for immediate resolution of a problem, limited resources available for changing the environment, a lack of appropriately trained staff in private residential homes, a shortfall of psychiatrists and a lack of input from clinical psychology and speech therapy. But, even with the use of optimum resources and good professional input, some behaviour problems remain unchanged, causing serious risk to the individual and others. In some individuals, the use of medication brings welcome relief to all concerned, such as the use of low doses of risperidone in those with autistic spectrum disorders, stereotypies and disturbed behaviour. In some, medication reduces arousal levels, allowing the individual to participate in other therapeutic approaches. Nevertheless, clinicians who use psychotropic drugs outside their licensed indications feel vulnerable and open to criticism for 'unethical practice'. Strong views exist about 'chemical straitjacketing' for behaviour disorders in the absence of adequate resources.

There is evidence that people with LD may handle drugs differently from the general population. Within the LD population, there is greater variation in the physical stature and physiological functioning among individuals than in the wider population. Such factors may result in different electrolyte and blood values, different volumes of distribution, and different renal and hepatic capacity.

These in turn may affect the pharmacokinetics and efficacy of a drug. The nature of the damage in the brain or changes in the brain structure that have given rise to the LD may result in:

- altered sensitivities to a drug
- changed effects of the drug
- difficulties in determining the optimum dose.

There is anecdotal evidence that people with LD experience more adverse drug reactions than the general population. However, studies show inconclusive results, possibly because of communication problems and reporting difficulties. Although there has been widespread concern about the use of antipsychotics, studies of the prevalence of tardive dyskinesia following long-term use of antipsychotics show mixed results. Guidelines for the use of psychotropic medication have been published in the *International Consensus Handbook*. It is also unclear whether there are specific drugs that present a greater benefit or hazard to adults with LD than adults in the general population, such as anticholinergics for dribbling, eye-drops, laxatives or hormone replacement therapy. Nevertheless, multiple health problems and consequent polypharmacy put individuals with LD at increased risk of adverse drug reactions and drug interactions.

These guidelines

The guidelines have been written in response to the above difficulties faced by clinicians. Their purpose is to allow a standardized practice across LD psychiatry, moving away from idiosyncratic prescribing toward a consensus approach based on both evidence and expert opinion.

However, every individual referred to LD psychiatric services is unique. Therefore, there may be considerable variation in the clinical approaches used. Hence this book has been produced as guidelines only and not as protocol.

The guidelines were written after a thorough examination of the current evidence base, followed by a series of peer reviews with clinicians (individually named in the Acknowledgements) from national clinical centres. The peer group included representatives from health districts in London and South-East Thames, the West Midlands and the Trent Region; Partnership in Care, Norfolk; the Academic Centre of the University of Birmingham; and the Neurology Services of the West Midlands. The current NICE guidelines in relevant areas have been incorporated where possible, including those for dementia, bipolar affective disorder and schizophrenia, with relevant modifications for those with LD.

The guidelines will be revised every 2 years. However, with the rapid growth and development of pharmacology and the continuing publication of NICE guidelines, readers are advised to keep abreast of recent developments and to modify the guidelines accordingly between publications. Updates are available in the publications section of the website **www.leicesterfrith.co.uk**.

These guidelines should not be used in isolation but should be seen as part of a holistic package of care that includes non-pharmacological approaches such as psychological input, community support, dealing with underlying physical problems and addressing environmental and social issues pertinent to the individual.

The core of real clinical improvement lies in a thorough understanding of the issues involved; empathy and rapport with service users and carers; and a thorough clinical assessment. It is these parameters that determine the success or failure of any treatment rather than a strict adherence to protocols or guidelines.

Disclaimer: no liability is accepted for any injury, loss or damage, however caused.

Key references

American Association on Mental Retardation. *Mental Retardation: Definition, Classification, and Systems of Supports.* Washington, DC: American Association on Mental Retardation, 1992.

British Medical Association and British Law Society. *Assessment of Medical Capacity. Guidance for Lawyers and Doctors.* London: British Medical Association, 1995.

Foundation for People with Learning Disabilities. *Learning Disabilities: The Fundamental Facts.* London: Mental Health Foundation, 2001.

Fryers T. *The Epidemiology of Severe Intellectual Impairment.* London: Academic Press, 1984.

General Medical Council. *Seeking Patients' Consent: The Ethical Considerations.* London: GMC, 1998.

Kalachnick JE, Leventhal BL, James DH et al. Guidelines for the use of psychotropic medication. In: Reiss S, Aman MG (eds). *Psychotropic Medications and Developmental Disabilities. The International Consensus Handbook.* Columbus, OH: Ohio State University Press, 1998, pp. 45–72.

McGrother CW, Thorp CF, Taub N, Machado O. Prevalence, disability and need in adults with severe learning disability. *Tizard Learning Disability Review* 2001; **6**: 236–271.

NHS Executive. *Good Practice in Consent.* Health Services Circular HSC 2001/203. London: Department of Health, 2001.

NHS Executive. *Seeking Consent: Working with People with Learning Disabilities.* Health Services Circular. London: Department of Health, 2001.

Russell O (ed). *Seminars in the Psychiatry of Learning Disabilities.* College Seminar Series. London: Royal College of Psychiatrists, Gaskell Press, 1997.

chapter 2

Epilepsy

Definition

Epilepsy is a condition characterized by recurrent (two or more) seizures unprovoked by an immediately identifiable cause. An epileptic seizure is a clinical manifestation presumed to result from an abnormal and excessive discharge of a set of neurons in the brain. Some specialists consider that a single seizure associated with electroencephalogram (EEG) changes may have a high chance of recurrence and should therefore be included in the definition of epilepsy.

The classification of seizures depends on whether the onset of the seizure begins locally or not, and on the nature of other symptoms and signs occurring during the seizure (Table 2.1). The distinction between simple and complex seizures based on whether consciousness is impaired or not during a seizure is contentious; the two are not easily distinguishable, particularly in those with limited speech.

Table 2.1 International classification of seizures§

Partial (focal) seizures (begin locally)	Simple partial seizures (consciousness not impaired)	With motor signs, e.g. Jacksonian epilepsy (focal tonic spasm)
		With somatosensory or special sensory signs, e.g. visual, auditory, olfactory, gustatory
		With autonomic signs or symptoms, e.g. salivation, flushing, sweating, pallor
		With psychological symptoms, e.g. perceptual or mood changes
	Complex partial seizures (with impaired consciousness)	Beginning as a simple partial seizure (aura), progressing to impaired consciousness
		With impaired consciousness at outset: alone or with automatisms (psychomotor attacks), e.g. lip-smacking, chewing, semipurposeful behaviour
	Partial seizures evolving to secondarily generalized seizures	Simple partial seizures or complex partial seizures becoming tonic-clonic seizures
Generalized seizures (no local onset, bilaterally symmetrical)	Absence seizures (petit mal)	Typical absence seizures; 3/s spike-and-wave on EEG and 10–45-s lapse of consciousness
		Atypical absence seizures (often associated with an epileptic syndrome): 1–2.5/s spikes on EEG
	Myoclonic seizures	Sudden brief (<350 ms) stereotypical shock-like muscle contractions (any muscle group)
	Clonic seizures	Rhythmic or semirhythmic contractions of a group of muscles (any muscle group)

Tonic seizures | Brief seizures (usually <60 s): sudden onset of increased tone in extensor muscles

Tonic-clonic seizures (grand mal) | Generalized stiffening of flexor or extensor muscles (tonic phase) followed by generalized jerking of muscles (clonic phase)

Atonic seizures (drop attacks) | Sudden loss in muscle tone

Unclassified | Any other seizures that do not fit into the above categories

§ International League Against Epilepsy and Epileptic Syndromes, Commission on Classification, 1989.

Prevalence

Epilepsy is a common condition. Studies in the general population show that the incidence rate is 50–120 per 100 000 people a year. The highest incidence rates are observed in babies and young children, and in older persons. The prevalence rate is 0.5–1.0% a year. The lifetime risk of an individual developing epilepsy is 3–5%.

There is a greater prevalence of epilepsy in those with learning disability (LD) than in the general population. The prevalence and the severity of seizures increase with the increasing degree of LD (Figure 2.1). Overall, 25% of individuals with LD have epilepsy, increasing to about 50% in those with severe/profound LD.

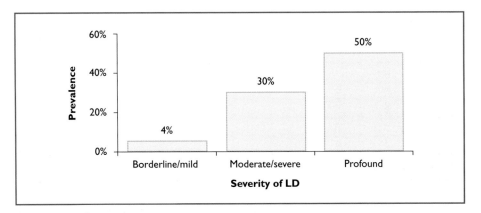

Figure 2.1 Prevalence of epilepsy in LD

If an individual with severe LD has seizures at the age of 22, there is a 40% probability of seizures having been present for over 10 years. This indicates how chronic a condition epilepsy can be in people with LD. The relationship between LD and epilepsy may be explained in a variety of ways.

Relationship between LD and epilepsy

- A brain abnormality leads to both LD and epilepsy, as in perinatal trauma, encephalopathy, head injury, non-accidental injury or neuromigrational defects.
- Seizures may rarely cause reduced IQ, as in febrile status and hypsarrhythmia.
- Treatment of epilepsy may reduce IQ, e.g. surgery or sedating drugs.
- Certain deteriorating conditions result in both reduced IQ and epilepsy, e.g. lipidoses, Sturge–Weber syndrome, tuberous sclerosis and disintegrative psychosis.

NB: Complex seizure status and non-convulsive generalized status may be mistaken for a low IQ and can continue to be unrecognized for long periods of time.

Aetiology

The causes of epilepsy may be genetic, congenital or acquired (Table 2.2). However, in many patients, the cause is unknown.

A genetic abnormality may result in epilepsy alone or in epilepsy with other neurological manifestations, as is found, for example, in Down syndrome and tuberous sclerosis. Many of the inborn errors of metabolism are associated with epilepsy. Most of these are very rare, and some, such as phenylketonuria and pyridoxine deficiency, are treatable. Susceptibility to intercurrent infections and a lowering of the seizure threshold by certain drugs may increase an individual's risk of developing epilepsy.

Table 2.2 Causes of epilepsy in people with LD

Classification	Examples
Genetic	
Chromosomal abnormalities	Down syndrome
Dysplastic conditions	Tuberous sclerosis Sturge–Weber syndrome Megalencephaly Aicardi's syndrome
Metabolic abnormalities	Phenylketonuria Maple syrup urine disease Pyridoxine deficiency Tay–Sachs disease Lipoidosis GM1 and GM3 Metachromatic leucodystrophy
Congenital	
Dysplastic and neoplastic conditions	Cortical dysplasia or dysgenesis Cerebral tumours
Vascular malformations	Atrial-ventricular malformation Cavernous angioma
Perinatal injury	Antenatal brain injury Perinatal brain injury
Acquired	
Trauma and injury	Head injury—dural tear, depressed fracture, intracranial bleed, anoxia Neurosurgery
Prenatal infections	Cytomegalovirus Syphilis Toxoplasmosis
Postnatal infections	Purulent meningitis Acute encephalitis Subacute sclerosing panencephalitis Postimmunization encephalopathy Post-traumatic infections
Metabolic disorders	Hepatic and renal disorders Hypoglycaemia and hyperglycaemia Hypocalcaemia and hypercalcaemia Anoxia
Toxic disorders	Alcohol or substance misuse Toxic effects of pharmacotherapy Lead
Vascular disease	Atherosclerosis Cardiovascular accident

Table 2.2 *Continued*

Classification	Examples
Hippocampal sclerosis	? Febrile convulsions in childhood
Neurological degenerative disease	Dementia
Tumours and other space-occupying lesions	Cerebral tumours Cerebral abscesses
Autistic syndromes associated with epilepsy	Rett syndrome Sturge–Weber syndrome

Certain causes of epilepsy are particularly likely to be related to the development of epilepsy from childhood. Other causes are more likely to be associated with the development of epilepsy in adolescence. Causes such as the development of dementia in people with Down syndrome may be associated with development of epilepsy even later in adulthood.

The commonest cause of most epilepsy in people with LD is developmental (Table 2.3). The brain passes though four main stages after the dorsal and ventral involutions of the embryonic neural plate, and at each there is the potential for abnormalities to develop.

Table 2.3 Pathogenesis of the developmental causes of epilepsy

Developmental process	Peak period	Results of abnormalities	Examples
Neuronal proliferation	2–4 months after conception	Microcephaly Macrocephaly	Tuberous sclerosis
Neuronal migration	First 6 months of gestation	Generalized focal abnormalities: pachygyria (gyri few and broad) polymicrogyria (excessive small gyri)	Heterotopia Agenesis of the corpus callosum
Neuronal organization	From month 6 of gestation to several years after birth	Abnormal neuronal organization Abnormal neuronal layering Abnormal ramification of nerves Abnormal synaptic proliferation	Rubella Phenylketonuria Down syndrome West syndrome

Table 2.3 *Continued*

Developmental process	Peak period	Results of abnormalities	Examples
Myelination	From month 3 of gestation to maturity	Abnormal myelination	Inborn errors of metabolism Infections Toxins Alcohol Hypoxia Hypoglycaemia

Key points specific to learning disability

Investigation

Clinical diagnosis is based on the following hierarchy of investigations.

Hierarchy of investigations for epilepsy in adults with LD

- seizure history
- seizure observation
- seizure registration (video)
- postictal/interictal electroencephalogram (EEG)
- postictal prolactin levels
- ambulatory monitoring of ictal EEG (with video if possible)
- telemetered EEG monitoring of ictal EEG (with video)
- telemetered EEG monitoring of ictal EEG (with video) using invasive electrodes (this is not without risk and is usually reserved for those for whom surgery is being considered).

Epilepsy is often difficult to diagnose in individuals with LD. They often have disordered cerebral anatomy or other cerebral disorders, which may alter the presentation of epilepsy. People with LD often lack the ability to give a subjective account of their seizures. For these reasons, good-quality cerebral imaging, such as magnetic resonance imaging (MRI), may also be useful. EEG and MRI can be offered to people with LD by well-trained staff, with the support of aids such as domiciliary EEG monitoring or echo planer MRI, where it is available, and sedation or light anaesthesia, where it is not.

The following other phenomena that occur in this population may be mistaken for epilepsy:

- severe, persistent EEG abnormalities (often mislabelled 'status epilepticus')
- dystonias, rocking, head movements such as nodding
- tongue thrusting
- abnormal postural reflexes (opisthotonus) or tonic neck reflex
- stereotypical behaviours, including chewing, buccal and autistic behaviours
- eye movements, eye deviation and nystagmus
- respiratory phenomena such as tachypnoea, apnoea and periodic breathing
- startle phenomena
- non-epileptic myoclonic phenomena
- sleep phenomena such as Sandifer's syndrome.

Epilepsy and autism

One-third of individuals with autism develop epilepsy during adolescence. This may be because autism is the final presentation of a variety of abnormalities of brain development and dysfunction that are also seen in people with epilepsy. No specific epileptic syndrome is evident with autism, although there are syndromal associations such as tuberous sclerosis, Sturge–Weber syndrome and Rett syndrome.

Epilepsy and Down syndrome

Approximately 10% of adults with Down syndrome have epilepsy, increasing to 40% of those over the age of 40 and to 80% of those with Alzheimer's disease.

There are three peaks in the incidence of epilepsy during the life span of an individual with Down syndrome:

- In early childhood, there is a particular association between epilepsy and West syndrome. In those with Down syndrome, West syndrome is more benign, with more myoclonic seizures and these more easily controlled than in those without Down syndrome.

- During the third decade of life, a rise in epilepsy among people with Down syndrome appears to be the equivalent of the increased incidence of partial epilepsies seen in adolescent individuals without LD. This is thought to be related to the myelination and proliferation of a sufficient bulk of nerves and synapses to connect abnormal areas of brain and thus allow paroxysmal spread.

- Epilepsy in Down syndrome finally peaks with the development of Alzheimer's disease in those over the age of 40. In 60% of individuals, seizures start after the clinical onset of dementia. The seizures are usually tonic-clonic, although myoclonic seizures may be particularly prominent. Interictal EEGs often show only non-specific slow-wave changes.

In addition to these increased incidences of epilepsy in Down syndrome, certain forms of epilepsy are less common than might be expected. For example, despite the increased incidence of infections in infants with Down syndrome, febrile convulsions are rare. There is also a lower incidence of Lennox–Gastaut syndrome, an important cause of severe epilepsy in people with LD.

The mechanisms by which epilepsy is generated in Down syndrome are not entirely clear, although it has been suggested that the following characteristics of the brain are relevant:

- small brain with abnormal neocortical cytoarchitecture

- reduced number of granule cells—possibly inhibitor GABA (gamma-aminobutyric acid) cells

- abnormal morphology of neurons and dendrites—this may enhance excitability

- altered neuronal physiology and membrane reactivity

- neurotransmitter abnormalities of 5-HT (5-hydroxytryptamine or serotonin) and glutamate.

There are a variety of causes of 'funny turns' in people with Down syndrome, including breath-holding, behaviour disturbance, heart dysrhythmia, sleep disorders and many undiagnosable episodes. Therefore, careful assessment with observation EEG and scanning is vital. If epilepsy is diagnosed, treatment is often effective.

Epilepsy and behaviour disorders

Behaviour problems are not uncommon in people with LD and active epilepsy. Often these behaviours have other causative factors such as maladaptive learned behaviour or interictal major mental health problems. For a significant minority, however, the behaviours may be directly linked to the epileptic activity.

These behaviours may occur preictally (aura), ictally (as in temporal lobe epilepsy) or during a postictal confusional state. Rarely, prolonged ictal activity, such as an atypical absence, may present entirely as a behaviour problem. Ideally, ambulatory EEG monitoring should be used to confirm the diagnosis.

Epilepsy and behaviour disorders will be covered in further detail in Chapter 3, which deals with organic mental disorders.

Multiple seizure types

Many people with LD and seizures experience more than one type of seizure. One study of an adult population with LD and seizures found that only 46% suffered from a single type of seizure. Although tonic-clonic seizures were the most common, absence seizures and myoclonic jerks occurred more frequently than in the general population with epilepsy.

Treatment

Goals of pharmacotherapy

The main goals of the drug treatment of epilepsy are as follows:

- to achieve control of or, ideally, freedom from seizures
- to maintain a quality of life that allows the individual to participate meaningfully in day-to-day activities.

These two goals need to be balanced, as full control of seizures is not always possible.

Good recording of seizures

Pivotal to good pharmacotherapy, it is important to have good recording systems in place, including the following features:

- clear descriptions of the various types of seizures in simple language rather than in medical terms
- clear recording of the frequency of each type of seizure type
- clear descriptions of how other aspects of the person's activities or behaviours have changed with the introduction of a new drug.

Choice of antiepileptics

The choice of antiepileptic drugs (AEDs) depends on the type of seizure (Table 2.4). Although a number of new AEDs have been introduced, carbamazepine and sodium valproate are still advocated by the National Institute for Clinical Excellence (NICE) as the drugs of first choice. However, sodium valproate should be avoided in women who may become pregnant. Carbamazepine is a high enzyme inducer and may therefore interact with other drugs; oxcarbamazepine may be an acceptable substitute.

Table 2.4 Drug treatment for different types of epilepsy in adults with LD

Type of seizure	First-line drugs	Second-line drugs
Partial seizures		
Simple partial seizures	Carbamazepine	Oxcarbazepine
Complex partial seizures	Sodium valproate	Gabapentin
Partial seizures evolving	Lamotrigine	Tiagabine
to secondarily generalized	Topiramate	Levetiracetam
seizures		
Generalized seizures		
Absence seizures (petit mal)	Sodium valproate	Ethosuximide
	Lamotrigine	
Myoclonic seizures	Sodium valproate	Lamotrigine
		Clonazepam
Tonic seizures	Sodium valproate	Clonazepam
Atonic seizures (drop attacks)	Lamotrigine	
	Topiramate	
Tonic-clonic seizures (grand mal)	Sodium valproate	Levetiracetam
	Carbamazepine	
	Lamotrigine	
	Topiramate	

Concerns remain about the toxicity of phenobarbital and phenytoin and their impact on behaviour. This makes these drugs unsuitable for the treatment of epilepsy in people with LD. Phenobarbital and phenytoin should only be used:

● when attempts to replace them have failed

● as a last resort.

Primidone presents similar problems and will shortly be withdrawn from clinical practice.

Polypharmacy

The refractory nature of seizures in many people with LD frequently results in polypharmacy of AEDs. For many, the introduction of new AEDs may result in increased polypharmacy with only marginal impact on seizures. For most people, it is unlikely that significant additional benefit will be achieved with more than two standard AEDs. If an AED has failed to produce significant benefits, the introduction of another AED should be followed by a gradual withdrawal of the first drug unless a synergistic effect is expected.

Side effects of antiepileptic drugs

The general side effects caused by most AEDs comprise:

● drowsiness

- dizziness

- ataxia

- gastrointestinal disturbances

- behaviour disturbances, including agitation, aggression and activation of psychosis.

In addition, individual drugs have a range of **specific side effects** (Table 2.5).

All drugs are more likely to cause side effects in the LD population. Therefore, it is advisable to start with a small dose, increase this gradually if necessary and avoid using a higher dose than necessary.

Table 2.5 Main side effects of specific antiepileptic drugs

Antiepileptic drug	Side effects	Comments
Carbamazepine	● Blurred vision, dizziness, unsteadiness	Dose-related; reduced by using modified-release drugs
	● Mild transient generalized erythematous rash	Withdraw drug if this worsens or if other symptoms present
	● Stevens–Johnson syndrome	Withdraw drug
Oxcarbazepine	● Blood dyscrasia: leucopenia, agranulocytosis, aplastic anaemia	Withdraw drug
	● Induction of hepatic enzymes: carbamazepine—potent inducer oxcarbazepine—less potent inducer	Lowers plasma concentration of — oral contraceptives — sodium valproate — ethosuximide — clonazepam
	● Hyponatraemia, oedema, disturbed bone metabolism	With osteomalacia
Ethosuximide	● Gastrointestinal symptoms common such as nausea ● Hiccoughs ● Sedation, headache ● Significantly higher risk of acute psychiatric reactions following seizure control (forced normalization) than with other anti-absence drugs including sodium valproate	
Clobazam	● Significant toxicity: sedation, dizziness, ataxia, diplopia	Reported in 85% patients Notable in 5–15% of them
	● Tolerance of the anticonvulsant effect and withdrawal symptoms	

Table 2.5 *Continued*

Antiepileptic drug	Side effects	Comments
Clonazepam		• Drowsiness, ataxia, incoordination
		• Behavioural and personality changes: hyperactivity, restlessness, short attention span, irritability, disruptiveness, aggressiveness
		• Nystagmus, dizziness, hypotonia, blurred vision, diplopia, psychotic reaction
		• Increased frequency of seizures and emergence of different types of seizures
Gabapentin		• Drowsiness, fatigue, dizziness are common
		• Increased frequency of seizures, especially deterioration of myoclonus
		• Increase in behaviour problems such as hyperactivity, unprovoked outbursts of anger
		• No idiosyncratic or hypersensitivity reactions or hepatotoxicity reported
Lamotrigine		• Headache, diplopia, dizziness, ataxia, tremor are common
		• Rash occurs in 3–5% of patients, necessitating withdrawal of drug
		• Rarely, Stevens–Johnson syndrome and erythema multiforme have been reported
		• Low incidence of sedation
Levetiracetam		• Undue sedation, irritability and aggression in a small proportion of those who take it
Topiramate		• Somnolence, dizziness, ataxia, psychomotor slowing, speech disorder, nervousness, nystagmus, paraesthesia
		• Emotional lability with mood disorders including depression
		• Altered behaviour, including psychotic symptoms
		• Hypersalivation, taste disorder
		• Adverse effect on cognition such as difficulty in word finding
Sodium valproate		• Weight gain in 50% patients; often nausea, vomiting, epigastric dizziness, diarrhoea
		• Drowsiness; sometimes postural tremor, nystagmus; rarely, incoordination, ataxia
		• Idiosyncratic reactions such as hyperammonaemia, pancreatitis
		• Mild transient elevation of hepatic enzymes commonly, less common hepatotoxicity may be dose-related or idiosyncratic
		• Altered behaviour, including psychotic symptoms
		• Anovulatory cycles, amenorrhoea, polycystic ovaries in women treated before age 20
Tiagabine		• Dizziness and some central nervous system effects
		• Minimal adverse effect on cognition

Refractory epilepsy

Refractory epilepsy is the presence of seizures despite the use of optimal drug therapy. In the general population, approximately 20–30% of people with active epilepsy suffer from refractory epilepsy. The incidence is higher in those with LD. Refractoriness of seizures varies according to the underlying and concomitant conditions. For example, a 12-year follow-up study found that 79% of those with epilepsy and LD alone became seizure-free (the same proportion as the general population), whereas only 39% of those with brain disorders in addition to seizures and LD became seizure-free. Individuals with epilepsy and a history of cerebral palsy often have an early onset of seizures that are poorly controlled.

Neurosurgery is the final option for those with severe refractory seizures. This includes focal resections, temporal lobectomy, multilobar resections, hemispherectomy and functional procedures such as multiple subpial transection, vagal nerve stimulation and corpus callosectomy. A substantial proportion of patients with LD improve after surgery, and some become totally seizure-free. However, the risk–benefit ratio of surgery must be assessed on an individual basis.

Interactions between antiepileptic drugs

Table 2.6 describes commonly encountered and known significant interactions between AEDs.

Table 2.6 Significant interactions known to occur between antiepileptic drugs

Drugs causing interaction	Drugs affected by interaction												
	CBZ	CLB	CLN	ESM	GBP	LTG	LEV	PB	PHT	PRM	TGB	TOP	VPA
Carbamazepine (CBZ)	–	NE	↓CLN	↓ESM	NE	↓LTG	NE	↑↓PB	↑↑PHT	↓PRM	↓TGB	↓TOP	↓VPA
Clobazam (CLB)	NE	–	NE	NE	NE	NE	NE	NE	NE	NE	NE	NE	↑VPA
Clonazepam (CLN)	↓CBZ	NE	–	NE	NE	NE	NE	NE	↓↑PHT	NE	NE	NE	NE
Ethosuximide (ESM)	NE	NE	NE	–	NE	NE	NE	NE	NE	NE	NE	NE	NE
Gabapentin (GBP)	NE	NE	NE	NE	–	NE	NE	NE	NE	NE	NE	NE	NE
Lamotrigine (LTG)	↑CBZ	NE	NE	NE	NE	–	NE	NE	NE	NE	NE	NE	NE
Levetiracetam (LEV)	NE	NE	NE	NE	NE	NE	–	NE	NE	NE	NE	NE	NE
Phenobarbital (PB)	↓CBZ	NE	↓CLN	↓ESM	NE	↓LTG	NE	–	↓↑PHT	NE	↓TGB	↓TOP	↓VPA
Phenytoin (PHT)	↓CBZ	NE	NE	↓ESM	NE	↓LTG	NE	↓↑PB	–	NE	↓TGB	↓TOP	↓VPA
Primidone (PRM)	↓CBZ	NE	↓CLN	↓ESM	NE	↓LTG	NE	NE	↓↑PHT	–	↓TGB	↓TOP	↓VPA
Tiagabine (TGB)	NE	NE	NE	NE	NE	NE	NE	NE	NE	NE	–	NE	NE
Topiramate (TOP)	NE	NE	NE	NE	NE	NE	NE	↓PB	NE	NE	NE	–	NE
Sodium valproate (VPA)	↑CBZ	NE	NE	↑ESM	NE	↑LTG	NE	↑PB	↑↓PHT	NE	NE	NE	–

NE: no interaction expected (in most cases); ↑: increased drug level of specified drug; ↓: decreased drug level of specified drug.

Key references

Betts T. *Epilepsy, Psychiatry and Learning Difficulty.* London: Martin Dunitz and Parthenon, 1998.

Betts T, Greenhill L. *Managing Epilepsy with Women in Mind.* London: Martin Dunitz and Parthenon, 2004.

Bronson LD, Wranne L. Long term prognosis in childhood epilepsy; survival and seizure prognosis. *Epilepsia* 1987; **28**: 324–330.

Commission on Classification and Terminology of the International League Against Epilepsy. Proposal for revised classification of epilepsies and epileptic syndromes. *Epilepsia* 1989; **30**: 389–399.

Deb S. Epilepsy and mental retardation. *Epilepsia Bulletin* 1987; **25**: 91–94.

Goulden J, Shinnar S, Koller H, Katz M, Richardson SA. Epilepsy in children with mental retardation: a cohort study. *Epilepsia* 1991; **32**: 690–697.

Isojarvi JIT, Tokola RA. Benzodiazepine in the treatment of epilepsy in people with intellectual disability. *Seizure* 1998; **7**: 509–512.

Kirkham F. Epilepsy and mental retardation. In: Hopkins A, Shorvon S, Cascmo G (eds). *Epilepsy.* London: Chapman & Hall Medical, 1995, pp. 503–520.

McVicker R, Shanks OEP, McClelland R. Prevalence and associated features of epilepsy in adults with Down's syndrome. *British Journal of Psychiatry* 1994; **164**: 528–532.

Shepherd C, Hosking G. Epilepsy in schoolchildren with intellectual impairment in Sheffield; the size and nature of the problem and its implications in service provision. *Journal of Mental Deficiency Research* 1989; **33**: 511–514.

chapter 3

Organic mental disorders

Definition

Organic mental disorders encompass a range of behaviour disorders with an organic or bio-logical aetiology. They include delirium, dementia, amnestic disorders, disorders arising from structural brain disease, epilepsy and psychiatric disorders caused by systemic disease arising outside the brain such as endocrine disease (ICD-10, DSM-IV). More than one condition may be present, resulting in a complex clinical picture. Where more than a single disorder exists or is suspected, it is important to differentiate symptoms and associated conditions of each disorder and to document the chronology of their appearance and development. This chapter focuses on individual disorders that are likely to produce behaviour symptoms within the learning disability (LD) population.

For the purposes of these treatment guidelines for adults with LD, organic mental disorders may be broadly classified into four categories:

- acute state of confusion or delirium

- seizure-related behaviour disorder

- behaviour disorder secondary to traumatic brain injury

- behaviour disorder as a symptom-complex of dementia of any aetiology.

Prevalence

The overall prevalence of organic brain disease in older people is difficult to estimate, although the risk factors have been shown to increase considerably with age. The prevalence of dementia in the general population over the age of 65 years is 2–7% for moderate and severe dementias, with greater variability for mild cases. The prevalence rises exponentially with age, doubling with each successive 5-year period. Studies show that the prevalence of dementia in older people with LD is considerably higher than in an age-matched sample from the general population. Within the LD population, 22% of those aged 65 and over have dementia. This drops to about 12% for those aged 50 and over, which is four times the prevalence for dementia in the age-matched general population.

Key points specific to learning disability

State of confusion or delirium

Co-morbid physical disabilities and medical disorders are very common in those with confusion/delirium and LD. Individuals with LD are also more likely to suffer from acute infections and fever because of a poorly developed immune system, and to experience toxic or withdrawal symptoms due to a low tolerance or altered metabolism of many therapeutic drugs. Metabolic disturbances, such as diabetic ketoacidosis, hypoglycaemia, hyponatraemia, hypernatraemia and hyperuricaemia, may be a significant cause of confusion/delirium. Iatrogenic factors, such as the introduction or rapid escalation of anticholinergic drugs and polypharmacy, may precipitate a delirium-like state (Table 3.1).

Table 3.1 Common causes of confusion/delirium in adults with LD

Classification	Examples
Drug intoxication	Anticholinergic drugs, antiepileptic drugs, steroids, digoxin, lithium, alcohol, illicit drugs
Drug withdrawal	Alcohol, benzodiazepines
Infections	Chest infections, urinary tract infections, septicaemia, meningitis
Metabolic disorders	Electrolyte disturbance: dehydration, water intoxication Uraemia, liver failure, respiratory failure, cardiac failure
Endocrine disorders	Diabetes mellitus: hypoglycaemia, hyperglycaemia, diabetic ketoacidosis Thyroid disease: hypothyroidism, hyperthyroidism
Nutritional deficiency	Deficiency of thiamine, nicotinic avid, vitamin B_{12}/folate
Central nervous system disorders	Transient ischaemic attacks Meningitis, encephalitis Any cause of increased intracranial pressure such as tumours
Epilepsy	Status epilepticus, postictal state
Head injury	Single or repeated

The management of an acute confusional state in people with LD is the same as for those in the general population. This comprises control of the environment; treatment of any underlying medical cause; and, if required, the judicious use of psychotropic drugs such as low doses of antipsychotics or benzodiazepines.

Seizure-related behaviour disorder

Behaviour disturbances are seen more frequently in people with epilepsy than in the general population. They are more common in temporal lobe epilepsy than in other forms of epilepsy, although many people with generalized seizures have behaviour disturbance. Behaviour disorders associated with seizures are classified as shown in the box.

	preictal	prodromal states and mood disturbance
Peri-ictal	ictal	complex partial seizures, absence status, complex partial status
	postictal	automatisms, impaired consciousness
Interictal		any psychiatric disorder such as schizophrenia or affective disorder

Two hypothetical mechanisms are postulated to explain the neurobiological correlation between epilepsy and behaviour disorder, kindling and forced normalization.

Kindling

Focal electrical stimulation of the brain results in an increase in neuronal excitability with the potential for 'after discharges' and spontaneous seizures. As kindling involves the spread of seizure activity from the site of stimulation to other areas of brain, it is a potential mechanism for the effects of focal epilepsy leading to behaviour disturbance.

Forced normalization

The neurochemical changes that promote epilepsy reduce the tendency to psychosis, and vice versa. Thus, there is said to be a 'biological antagonism' between epilepsy and schizophrenia. Some psychoses in epilepsy have been correlated with normalization of the electroencephalogram (EEG).

Seizures with motor agitation are a characteristic feature of frontal lobe epilepsy. These seizures involve motor activity that is both bizarre and violent. This may include thrashing and flailing of the limbs, vocalizations such as giggling and shouting, and prominent facial flushing. Frontal lobe seizures are often mistaken for pseudo-seizures, a non-epileptic attack disorder of psychogenic origin in which the individual mimics certain symptoms of an epileptic seizure. Pseudo-seizures can be differentiated from epilepsy on the basis of the setting, clinical presentation and EEG findings.

A full assessment of an individual with LD is essential before starting any medication aimed at behaviour modification. Antiepileptic drugs (AEDs), alone or when prescribed with other AEDs or other drugs, may induce or potentiate behaviour disturbance. The AEDs most frequently implicated in causing behaviour disturbance are phenobarbital, phenytoin and vigabatrin. Carbamazepine, sodium valproate and benzodiazepines may also cause disinhibition. Lamotrigine may cause behavioural impairment in those with LD and epilepsy.

AEDs may have a significant effect on cognitive function and behaviour, and the negative effects of these drugs on behaviour can be additive, even at therapeutic levels. Many studies demonstrate the beneficial effects of reducing AED polytherapy, including improvement in mood, behaviour, personality, psychomotor performance, concentration and memory.

Changes in behaviour may also be precipitated by interactions between AEDs and other drugs. Co-administration of psychotropic drugs, such as antidepressants or haloperidol and other antipsychotics, may alter behaviour. Calcium channel blockers, such as diltiazem and verapamil, may elevate plasma levels of carbamazepine.

Traumatic brain injury

Studies of head injuries in individuals with normal intelligence have shown the emergence of significant affective symptoms, personality changes and schizophrenia-like syndromes after the injury. In particular, an increase in depression, mania and mood lability (pathological laughing and crying) is observed in those with traumatic brain injury. Personality changes after brain trauma may be associated either with a lack of volition and apathy or with disinhibition, aggression and impulsivity. Irritability is extremely common in such individuals.

Schizophrenia-like syndromes following brain trauma occur more frequently in people with LD than in the general population. Studies have shown an association between psychosis and trauma to the temporal lobe.

Dementia

This section focuses on dementia syndromes: their overlap with behavioural psychiatric disturbances, salient issues related to their diagnosis, and pharmacological interventions to control the symptoms affecting an individual's quality of life such as aggression, inappropriate behaviour and sleep disturbance. Details of the specific dementias and dementia complexes are beyond the scope of this chapter.

Broadly, dementia may arise from a primary degenerative process or be secondary to a wide range of diseases or trauma (Table 3.2). Dementia syndromes are divided into cortical and subcortical groups, each with characteristic features, although there is considerable overlap between the two groups.

The association between Down syndrome and Alzheimer's disease is well known (and this is discussed further in Chapter 4, which deals with Down syndrome and dementia). Alzheimer's disease may also occur frequently in those with LD of other aetiologies.

People with LD and dementia but without Down syndrome have a similar increase in psychotic symptoms to people with dementia in the general population. In marked contrast, people with Down syndrome and dementia seldom show evidence of delusions and hallucinations but report significant mental symptoms that may be challenging to carers, such as difficulty with sleeping, hypersomnia, irritability, inefficient thought processes, social withdrawal and lassitude.

Deterioration in sensory function, thyroid abnormalities and seizures frequently occur at the same time as other symptoms of dementia. Depression may occur during the prodromal period that precedes the appearance of early cognitive changes associated with Alzheimer's disease and may be difficult to distinguish from the signs and symptoms of dementia per se.

Table 3.2 Outline of the causes and features of dementia

Classification		Examples	Features
Degenerative	Cortical	Alzheimer's disease Multi-infarct dementia Dementia of mixed type Pick's disease	Impairment of higher cerebral functions including perception, memory, language, integrated motor control: ● aphasia ● agnosia ● apraxia
		Dementia with Lewy bodies	Features of both cortical and subcortical syndromes plus specific characteristics: ● fluctuations in consciousness ● affective symptoms ● visual hallucinations ● sensitivity to antipsychotic drugs
	Subcortical	Parkinson's disease Huntington's chorea Progressive supranuclear palsy	More subtle cognitive decline: ● slowing rate of cognitive processing ● impaired executive function ● disordered mood
Secondary	Intracranial	Normal pressure hydrocephalus Subdural haematoma Tumours	
	Traumatic	Head injury	
	Infections and related conditions	Encephalitis Neurosyphilis Prion disease	
	Vascular	Vascular dementia Occlusion of the carotid artery	Features of subcortical dementia and of underlying cause
	Metabolic	Sustained uraemia	
	Endocrine	Hypothyroidism	
	Nutritional	Lack of vitamin B_{12}/folate or thiamine	
	Anoxia	Chronic respiratory failure Anaemia	
	Toxic	Alcohol or heavy metal poisoning	

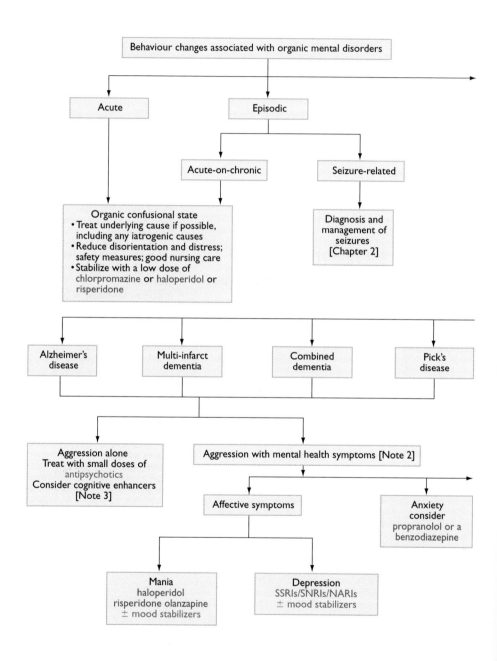

Behaviour changes associated with organic mental disorders

Acute

Episodic

Acute-on-chronic

Seizure-related

Organic confusional state
• Treat underlying cause if possible, including any iatrogenic causes
• Reduce disorientation and distress; safety measures; good nursing care
• Stabilize with a low dose of chlorpromazine or haloperidol or risperidone

Diagnosis and management of seizures
[Chapter 2]

Alzheimer's disease

Multi-infarct dementia

Combined dementia

Pick's disease

Aggression alone
Treat with small doses of antipsychotics
Consider cognitive enhancers
[Note 3]

Aggression with mental health symptoms [Note 2]

Affective symptoms

Anxiety consider propranolol or a benzodiazepine

Mania
haloperidol risperidone olanzapine
± mood stabilizers

Depression
SSRIs/SNRIs/NARIs
± mood stabilizers

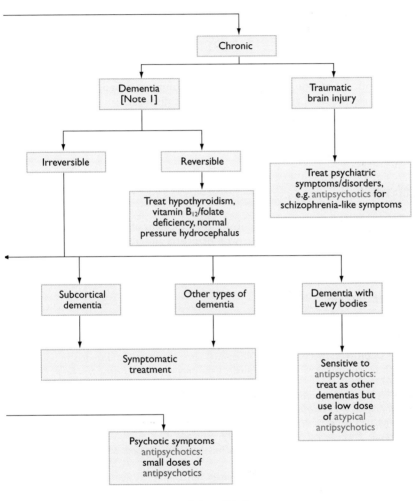

```
                              ┌──────────────────┐
                              │     Chronic      │
                              └──────────────────┘
              ┌──────────────────┐          ┌──────────────────┐
              │    Dementia      │          │    Traumatic     │
              │    [Note 1]      │          │   brain injury   │
              └──────────────────┘          └──────────────────┘
```

Irreversible   Reversible

Treat hypothyroidism,
vitamin B₁₂/folate
deficiency, normal
pressure hydrocephalus

Treat psychiatric
symptoms/disorders,
e.g. antipsychotics for
schizophrenia-like symptoms

Subcortical
dementia

Other types of
dementia

Dementia with
Lewy bodies

Symptomatic
treatment

Sensitive to
antipsychotics:
treat as other
dementias but
use low dose
of atypical
antipsychotics

Psychotic symptoms
antipsychotics:
small doses of
antipsychotics

NB: Committee on Safety of Medicines

1. There is an increased risk of cerebrovascular adverse events in older patients with dementia treated with olanzapine or risperidone.
2. Please refer to caution regarding the use of SSRIs and SNRIs.

Algorithm 3.1   Treatment of organic mental disorders in adults with LD

Note 1: *dementia.* Elderly people should be treated with caution due to changes in the body's rates of absorption, distribution, metabolism and excretion and the diminished physiological reserve that occurs with age. Thus, previously well-tolerated medications may produce acute side effects, and lower doses may be justified.

Note 2: *mental health symptoms.* Treatment of depression and psychiatric disorders in individuals with dementia and LD is paramount. Antidepressant drugs have most effect on those who are behaviourally non-compliant, or who have eating and sleeping disturbances or low energy levels. Antipsychotics need to be used cautiously, as they are more likely to produce dose-related neurological side effects, including dyskinesia and Parkinsonian symptoms in older people with LD and dementia. Mood-stabilizing drugs may be helpful in those with aggressive outbursts with affective instability that is not associated with depression. Sleep disturbance is common in people with dementia and can be a manifestation of an associated psychiatric disorder.

Note 3: *cognitive enhancers.* The use of antidementia drugs in the LD population, especially those with Down syndrome and Alzheimer's disease, is discussed in Chapter 4, which deals with Down syndrome.

Treatment

Algorithm 3.1 should be used as a guide only for the treatment of adults with both LD and organic mental disorders. For new patients with dementia and behaviour problems, follow the guidelines from the Faculty of Psychiatry of Old Age of the Royal College of Psychiatrists.

Key references

Bhaumik S, Branford D, Duggirala C, Ismail IA. A naturalistic study of the use of vigabatrin, lamotrigine and gabapentin in adults with learning disabilities. *Seizure* 1997; **6**: 127–133.

Collacott RA, Cooper S-A, McGrother C. Differential rates of psychiatric disorders in adults with Down's syndrome compared with other mentally handicapped adults. *British Journal of Psychiatry* 1992; **161**: 671–674.

Cooper S-A. Psychiatric symptoms of dementia amongst elderly people with learning disabilities. *International Journal of Geriatric Psychiatry* 1997; **12**: 662–666.

Cooper S-A. High prevalence of dementia among people with learning disabilities not attributable to Down syndrome. *Psychological Medicine* 1997; **27**: 609–616.

Lund J. The prevalence of psychiatric disorders in mentally retarded adults. *Acta Psychiatrica Scandinavica* 1985; **72**: 563–570.

Reynolds EH. Antiepileptic drugs and psychopathology. In: Trimble MR (ed). *Psychopharmacology of Epilepsy.* London: Wiley, 1985, pp. 49–63.

Royal College of Psychiatrists. Atypical antipsychotics and BPSD. Prescribing update (2004) for old age psychiatrists. At http://www.repsych.ac.uk/college/faculty/oap/BPSD.pdf

Shorvon S. Epilepsy arising in the frontal lobe. In: Shorvon S (ed). *Handbook of Epilepsy Treatment.* London: Blackwell Science, 2000, pp. 12–13.

Trimble MR. Kindling, epilepsy and behaviour. In: Bolwig T, Trimble MR (eds). *Clinical Relevance of Kindling.* Chichester: Wiley, 1989, pp. 177–190.

Wolf P. Acute behavioural symptomatology at disappearance of epileptiform EEG abnormality: paradoxical or 'forced' normalisation. In: Smith D, Treiman D, Trimble M (eds). *Advances in Neurology.* New York: Raven, 1991; vol. 55, pp. 127–142.

chapter 4

Down syndrome and dementia

Definition

Down syndrome is the most common cause of learning disability (LD), accounting for about 30% of all cases. Inheritance of an extra chromosome 21 after non-disjunction during miotic cell division is responsible for 95% of cases of Down syndrome. The non-disjunction is of maternal origin, and the risk increases with maternal age. The remaining 5% of cases are due to translocation, which may occur between the long arms of chromosomes 14 and 21— t(14q 21q)—or in chromosome 21. The phenotype mosaicism results from an individual's having two or more cell lines, one of which has a trisomy 21.

The mean life expectancy of people with Down syndrome is less than that of the general population. However, it has increased from a life span of less than 10 years in the early 1900s to almost 50 years more recently. Twenty per cent or more of people with Down syndrome may be over the age of 55 years at any one time. This improvement has made the prevalence of age-related health problems apparent. The most important of these is the risk of developing Alzheimer-like neuropathological change and dementia of the Alzheimer type.

Prevalence

The prevalence of Down syndrome is 1 in 660 live births.

The pathological relationship between Down syndrome and Alzheimer's disease has been recognized for many years. Studies show that 15–30% of people with Down syndrome develop Alzheimer's disease. The prevalence of Alzheimer's disease in people with Down syndrome aged 35–49 years is 8%. In those over 60 years of age, it is 50–75%.

Aetiology

The understanding of the aetiology of Alzheimer's disease in individuals with Down syndrome is currently fragmentary. Investigations have shown a longitudinal picture of the brain changes associated with the development of the classical neuropathological features of Alzheimer's disease. Five possible causative factors of Alzheimer's disease in people with Down syndrome have been identified.

Amyloid precursor protein

One of the defining characteristics of the neuropathology of Alzheimer's disease is the extracellular deposits of the amyloidogenic peptide β/A4 within nerve plaques in the brain. Studies of brain tissue of people with Down syndrome have shown that the deposition of β/A4 begins significantly earlier than it does in the general population. β/A4 is derived from a much larger precursor protein, the amyloid precursor protein (APP). It has been hypothesized that overexpression of APP in Down syndrome leads to the premature accumulation of β/A4. Point mutations in APP near the β/A4 domain have been more recently linked to Alzheimer's disease in a small number of familial cases. Although it does not appear that the mutations result in overexpression of APP, their presence supports the view that altered processing or stability of APP is important in the pathogenesis of Alzheimer's disease.

Superoxide dismutase

The distal segment of the long arm of chromosome 21 encodes the gene for cytoplasmic superoxide dismutase (SOD-1). The function of SOD-1 is thought to be the conversion of the superoxide anion to oxygen and hydrogen peroxide. A 50% increase in SOD-1 activity has been found in the cells of individuals with Down syndrome. The intracellular concentrations of SOD-1 and hydrogen peroxide are capable of pathological interaction with many structural cell elements such as proteins, lipids and polynucleotides. It has been postulated that SOD-1 overactivity might injure the brain in this way. However, there is no evidence of any Alzheimer-like neuropathology in the brains of transgenic mice that overexpress the human SOD-1 gene. The association between SOD-1 activity and the pathogenesis of Alzheimer's disease in Down syndrome is yet to be fully established.

Brain vulnerability

Specific brain regions appear to be selectively vulnerable in Alzheimer's disease: certain brainstem nuclei (locus coeruleus and raphe nuclei), basal forebrain, amygdala, hippocampus, entorhinal cortex and association areas of the neocortex. Within the basal forebrain, cholinergic neurons are particularly vulnerable. At least two studies have found that a significant decrease in the number of neurons in the basal forebrain of people with Down syndrome occurred before the appearance of other Alzheimer's disease neuropathology.

Premature ageing

It has been argued that Alzheimer's disease in people with Down syndrome may reflect one consequence of premature ageing. Although there is evidence of premature ageing in some organ systems of people with Down syndrome, this is not the case for all systems.

Genetic association

The frequency of Down syndrome increases in relatives of people with Alzheimer's disease. This led to the hypothesis that trisomy 21 cells accumulate over time by unequal chromosome segregation during mitosis in the brains of people with sporadic Alzheimer's disease. This could lead to the changes of Alzheimer's disease as seen in the brains of people with Down syndrome, but at a later age due to the modulating effects of mosaicism.

Key points specific to learning disability

Discrepancy between the onset of neuropathological and clinical changes

Although the excessive amyloid deposition, plaques and tangle formation of Alzheimer's disease appear in the brains of people with Down syndrome at a young age, most studies report that the mean age of clinical onset of Alzheimer's disease is in the early part of the fifth decade. Four reasons have been suggested for this discrepancy.

- Poor language skills may mask the subtle early changes of dementia such as memory difficulties.

- Although the majority of people with Down syndrome have significant intellectual impairment, they function within a considerable range of cognitive abilities, daily living activities and social skills. Thus, if an individual with Down syndrome declines in later life due to dementia, it may not be recognized as such but be attributed instead to the individual's intellectual disability. A reliable diagnosis can only be made if there is information available from long-standing carers about the individual's past ability. Subtle changes of cognitive decline may also be missed because of the high level of dependency on their carers.

- A pathological threshold to dementia may exist. For example, a critical level of cerebral amyloid deposition or of changes in protein may need to occur before the clinical symptoms of compromised cerebral function become apparent. Alternatively, an asymptomatic 'incubation period' of 10–20 years may be required before clinical signs can be observed.

- The healthy survivor effect proposes that all people with Down syndrome would eventually develop dementia if they lived long enough.

Diagnosis of Alzheimer's disease in people with Down syndrome

The diagnosis of dementia in individuals with Down syndrome requires evidence of a definitive change in those areas of cognitive functioning that are known to deteriorate with Alzheimer's disease. These include the development of impairments in memory, language ability (aphasia), ability to perform complex tasks (apraxia), orientation in time and place, daily living skills and personality (DSM-IV, ICD-10).

The objective measurement of cognitive function and the detection of any changes remain a challenge for clinicians. There are specific difficulties in the evaluation of individuals with LD by diagnostic criteria that are designed for people with normal intelligence and normal psychosocial functioning. Five factors are particularly limiting:

- A diminished ability to think abstractly and to communicate clearly may lead to difficulty in describing subjective symptoms.

- Impoverished social skills and life experiences may result in difficulties in identifying subtle clinical changes.

- The presentation may mimic an atypical picture of a psychiatric illness.

- Exacerbation of pre-existing cognitive deficits and challenging behaviours may create difficulties in establishing the onset of a newly developed disorder.

- Other disabilities, sensory impairments and problems with compliance with investigations such as magnetic resonance imaging may interfere with the diagnostic process.

A number of clinical problems may mimic dementia in those with Down syndrome. These disorders may coexist with dementia and require treatment.

Differential diagnosis of dementia

- depression
- life events such as bereavement
- hypothyroidism
- other physical illnesses
- sensory impairment
- a combination of the above.

Treatment

The management of behavioural and psychiatric symptoms in Alzheimer's disease is discussed in Chapter 3, which deals with organic mental disorders. The focus here is on antidementia drugs and the guidelines for their use in adults with LD and Alzheimer's disease according to the American Association of Mental Retardation (AAMR).

Antidementia drugs

The following antidementia drugs may be used in the early and mid stages of dementia:

- donepezil—a reversible acetylcholinesterase inhibitor (given once daily)

- galantamine—a dual mode of action: both a reversible acetylcholinesterase inhibitor and an allosteric potentiating ligand at nicotinic cholinergic receptors sites

- memantine—an NMDA-receptor antagonist (given twice daily)

- rivastigmine—a reversible non-competitive anticholinesterase inhibitor (given twice daily).

The investigation of the use of antidementia drugs such as donepezil, galantamine, memantine and rivastigmine in people with Alzheimer's disease and LD is still in its early stages. So far, there is no conclusive evidence that these drugs are efficacious. However, the general opinion is that they may improve the quality of life for patients and their carers.

There are a number of problems in translating the benefits of antidementia drugs observed in people with normal intelligence to those with LD. The key ones are as follows:

- establishing a clear diagnosis

- grading the dementia

- the lack of objective measures of the efficacy in the LD population and for recording adverse events.

Staging of dementia

The staging of dementia is understandably quite difficult in people with LD. The changes that are most notable vary according to the severity of the LD. For example, apathy, day-time drowsiness and loss of self-help skills are more evident in those with moderate LD. Deterioration of gait, myoclonus and seizures are more obvious in those with severe LD. Nevertheless, three broad clinical stages of dementia have been identified (Table 4.1).

Rating scales

A range of rating scales are available to assist in the diagnosis of dementia and to monitor changes in severity (Table 4.2).

Table 4.1 The clinical stages of dementia in people with LD

Stage	Main features	Use of antidementia drugs
Early	• Disorientation • Memory impairment • Deterioration of activities of daily living	Most likely to be effective at this stage
Mid	• Progressive loss of verbal and motor skills • Significant deterioration in the level of functioning • Changes in personality: loss of usual affectionate responses to others tendency to be hyperkinetic or impulsive withdrawal automatic speech • Emergence of psychiatric symptoms: hallucinations delusions mood changes aggression	May show limited effectiveness
Late	• Bladder/bowel incontinence • Mutism • Gait disturbance with frequent falls • Myoclonus • Seizures	Unlikely to provide any benefit

Adverse effects

The significant side effects of antidementia drugs include:

- gastrointestinal disturbances: nausea, vomiting, diarrhoea, abdominal pain; rarely, gastrointestinal haemorrhage

- cardiovascular effects: dizziness, syncope, bradycardia; rarely, sinoatrial and AV (atrio-ventricular) block (especially with donepezil)

- urinary incontinence, with the potential of bladder outflow obstruction

- convulsions.

These are cholinergic effects, which are dose-related. They can be minimized by starting treatment at a low dose and increasing it gradually according to the response.

Figure 4.1 should be used as a guide only for the treatment of dementia in adults with LD resulting from Down syndrome.

Table 4.2 Key rating scales used in dementia

Purpose	Rating scale	Brief description	Administered by
To establish a diagnosis	DC-LD	A modifed version of the Schedules for Clinical Assessment in Neuropsychiatry (SCAN)	Trained clinicians
	ICD-10	A classificatory system providing operationalized diagnostic criteria; used with ICD-10 manual	
	Visser's early dementia checklist	37 items covering cognitive and social functions. Diagnosis made if 12 items scored positively	Carers
	Dementia questionnaire for Mentally Retarded Persons (DMR)	50 items in eight subscales include: ● short-term and long-term memory ● orientation in time and space ● speech ● mood ● behaviour disturbance ● practical skills ● activities and interests Diagnosis if oval cognitive scores increase by 9 points or if total score increases by 13	Carers
To monitor the impact of treatment	Adaptive Behaviour Scale (ABS) Part I	Measures personal independence (Part I) and social skills (Part II) to give domain, factor and comparison scores	Trained clinicians
	Vineland Adaptive Behaviour Scale (Interview edition)	Covers four domains: communication, daily living skills, socialization and motor skills	Trained clinicians
	Relatives Stress Scale	14-item scale that measures stress among the relatives caring for the affected individual	Care worker
	Aberrant Behaviour Checklist	58-item scale administered to staff or carer	Trained clinicians

Diagnosis of probable Alzheimer's disease in adults with LD and Down syndrome:
• exclude other causes of dementia (Table 3.1), especially vascular dementia, depression, effects of sensory impairment and treatable causes of dementia
• check thyroid function
• if possible, arrange for MRI or CT scan
• consider using DC-LD or ICD-10 diagnostic criteria (Table 4.2)

↓

If Alzheimer's disease is in the early or mid stages, **consider using antidementia drugs** following the AAMR guidelines:
• consider the risks and benefits of treatment with antidementia drugs
• discuss the risks and benefits with users/carers
• gain user/carer consent for a trial of treatment and ensure compliance with medication
• carry out electrocardiogram (ECG) if necessary

↓

Identify key problem areas using one or more of the following scales:
• Dementia questionnaire for Mentally Retarded Persons (DMR)
• Adaptive Behaviour Scale (ABS) Part I
• Vineland Adaptive Behaviour Scale (Vineland)
• Relatives Stress Scale (RSS) (Table 4.2)
• Aberrant behaviour checklist (ABC)

↓

Begin treatment with donepezil, galantamine, rivastigmine or memantine at the minimum possible dose
Monitor closely for any adverse drug reactions—establish telephone link with carers

↓

Reassess the patient in clinic after 4 weeks:
• efficacy of treatment, especially in key problem areas
• any serious adverse drug reactions; stop drugs
• consider increasing the dose if needed

↓

Continue to monitor closely for:
• clinical improvement
• any adverse drug reactions

↓

Reassess clinically at end of 12 weeks and 24 weeks:
• reassess key problem areas using DMR, ABS Part I, Vineland or RSS or ABC
• stop drug treatment in those who show no benefit

↓

Continue treatment in those who show benefit and reassess at the end of 48 weeks:
reassess key problem areas using DMR, ABS Part I, Vineland or RSS or ABC

↓

If treatment is continued beyond 48 weeks:
• continue to monitor patient at 6-month intervals using the rating scales
• advise carers about reasons for possible discontinuation of treatment in the future such as progression to late stage of the disease

Algorithm 4.1   Diagnosis and treatment of dementia in adults with LD and Down syndrome

Key references

American Association of Mental Retardation: Rush AJ, Frances A (eds). Expert consensus guideline series. *American Journal of Mental Retardation* 2000; **105**: 159–227.

Evenhuis HM. The natural history of dementia in Down's syndrome. *Archives of Neurology* 1990; **47**: 263–267.

Mann DMA. Association between Alzheimer disease and Down syndrome: neuropathological observations. In: Berg JM, Karlinsky H, Holland AJ (eds). *Alzheimer's Disease, Down Syndrome and Their Relationship*. Oxford: Oxford University Press, 1993, pp. 71–92.

Oliver C, Holland AJ. Down's syndrome and Alzheimer's disease: a review. *Psychological Medicine* 1986; **16**: 307–322.

Potter H. Review and hypothesis: Alzheimer's disease and Down syndrome—chromosome 21 nondisjunction may underlie both disorders. *American Journal of Human Genetics* 1992; **48**: 1192–1200.

Prasher VP, Huxley A, Hague MS; Down Syndrome Ageing Study Group. A 24-week, double-blind, placebo-controlled trial of donepezil in patients with Down syndrome and Alzheimer's disease: a pilot study. *International Journal of Geriatric Psychiatry* 2002; **17**: 270–278.

Sovner R. Limiting factors in the use of DMS-III criteria with mentally ill/mentally retarded persons. *Psychopharmacology Bulletin* 1986; **22**: 1055–1059.

Zigman W, Schupf N, Havernan M et al. Epidemiology of Alzheimer's disease in mental retardation: results and recommendations from an international conference—Washington, DC: American Association on Mental Retardation. *Journal of Intellectual Disability Research* 1995; **41**: 76–80.

chapter 5

Self-injurious behaviour

Definition

Self-injurious behaviour (SIB) or self-mutilation is the deliberate alteration or destruction of body tissue without conscious suicidal intent. It may be viewed as a symptom of a psychiatric disorder or as a distinct syndrome.

SIB is classified into three types:

- major—severe self-mutilation seen in acute psychiatric illness or severe personality disorder

- superficial—less severe self-mutilation commonly associated with many psychiatric conditions

- stereotypic—self-mutilation seen mostly in institutionalized adults with learning disability (LD) or those with antistic disorders.

SIB commonly presents with:

- self-striking such as face-slapping and head-banging

- biting various parts of the body

- pinching, scratching, poking or pulling various parts of the body as in eye-poking and hair-pulling.

The following guidelines will focus on SIB in relation to LD in the context of behaviour arising from maladaptive learning or in association with behavioural phenotypes.

SIB is symptomatic of many underlying causes, including communication difficulties, physical health problems and pain. Clinically significant SIB presents serious challenges to professionals and may cause severe distress to carers. SIB may also reduce an individual's quality of life, as by exclusion from community-based educational facilities or day services.

Prevalence

The point prevalence of SIB differs between studies depending on the definition of SIB, the methodology used and the population studied. A prevalence of 1.7–41% has been reported in adults with LD, with 4.2–16% in community-based studies.

Although SIB is well documented in two X-linked conditions—Lesch–Nyhan syndrome and fragile X syndrome—there is no significant difference in the overall prevalence of SIB between the sexes. The prevalence of SIB shows a curvilinear relationship with age, being more common in adolescents and young adults than in children or older people. There appears to be a direct relationship between SIB and severity of LD (Figure 5.1). SIB has also been reported more frequently in people who are blind or have speech problems or autistic spectrum disorder. It has been associated with genetic conditions such as Cornelia de Lange syndrome, Prader–Willi syndrome, Rett syndrome and Smith–Magenis syndrome.

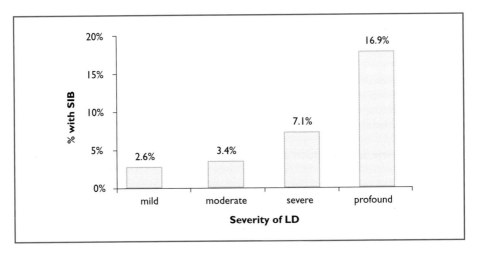

Figure 5.1　Prevalence of SIB by severity of LD

Aetiology

The heterogeneous nature of SIB has led to a number of aetiological theories. The main ones comprise SIB as a learned behaviour (behavioural model), SIB being due to a neuro-chemical imbalance (biological model), and SIB as part of grief or a psychiatric disorder such as depression or post-traumatic stress. SIB may occur as a symptom of acute organic illness (otitis media), chronic organic illness (epilepsy) or intermittent physical discomfort (menstruation). It may result from self-stimulation in a person with sensory deficit or hypersensitivity to sensory input, or be a part of stereotypies. SIB may also be a form of communication or compulsive behaviour.

Behavioural model

Behavioural theories are based on operant conditioning (where the frequency of the behaviour depends on the response to that behaviour). A number of subtypes have been identified (Table 5.1). A detailed functional analysis is essential when evaluating SIB.

Table 5.1 Behavioural subtypes of SIB	
Behavioural mechanism	**Prevalence**
Positive reinforcement by attention	27%
Positive reinforcement by tangible items	3%
Negative reinforcement by escape avoidance of demands	38%
Reinforcement by sensory consequences	21%
Multiple functions	5%

Biological model

The biological model is based on three types of neurotransmitters: dopamine, opioids and serotonin.

Dopamine

Responses to dopamine agonists, such as pemoline, and findings in Lesch–Nyhan syndrome lend support to the dopamine receptor oversensitivity theory. D_1-receptors are thought to be the principal dopamine receptors involved, a concept with therapeutic implications, since many traditional antipsychotics have little effect at these sites. Newer antipsychotics, such as olanzapine and clozapine, are more active at these receptors and have reportedly been successful in treating SIB in some individuals.

Opioids

Studies showing raised plasma beta-endorphin levels in people with SIB, or a reduction in SIB in response to administration of opiate-blocking agents, support the involvement of endogenous opiates. However, it is unclear whether SIB is the cause or an effect of raised endogenous opiates.

Serotonin

Low levels of serotonin have been found in people with Cornelia de Lange syndrome and SIB. Case reports suggest a treatment response to selective serotonin re-uptake inhibitors (SSRIs), such as fluoxetine, and tricyclic antidepressants, such as clomipramine.

Biomedical model

In practice, a combination of the above theories and other factors, such as expressive communication problems, may influence both the susceptibility to and type of SIB. In the biomedical model, a number of subtypes of SIB are identified, each with an emphasis on a specific neurotransmitter system (Table 5.2).

Key points specific to learning disability

Assessment

Assessment should take account of all the aetiological features outlined above unless an obvious remediable cause explains the behaviour, Assessment should be multidisciplinary since a combination of approaches is more likely to succeed than a single one.

Behavioural programmes

In view of the possibility of serious drug side effects, a behaviour programme should be tried before introducing medication. A behaviour-monitoring programme should remain in place during treatment with psychotropic medication. This should include systematic direct observations and, in special cases, the use of rating scales such as the Aberrant Behaviour Checklist or Self-injury Trauma Scale.

Clinical subtypes of self-injurious behaviour

With a biomedical model, clinical subtypes are determined by the presence of certain clinical features (Table 5.2).

The treatment of choice depends on the subtype of SIB (Table 5.2). The drug treatment of SIB should be used after behavioural methods and other approaches have been tried. Some people who display predominantly pain insensitivity benefit from opiate antagonists. Low doses of typical or atypical antipsychotics may be useful for autistic individuals displaying stereotypies and challenging SIB. Where a compulsive element is suspected, SSRIs, such as fluoxetine 40 mg or paroxetine 20 mg, or a tricyclic antidepressant, such as clomipramine, may be useful. Individuals with high levels of anxiety or arousal often respond to mood-stabilizing drugs or propranolol. Certain syndromal associations may need a different approach to control the SIB.

Treatment

Algorithm 5.1 should be used as a guide only for treatment of adults with both LD and SIB.

Table 5.2 Clinical subtypes of SIB (based on a biomedical model)

Subtype	Key feature	Inclusion criteria	Neurotransmitter system	Treatment
Extreme self-inflicted tissue damage	Pain insensitivity	Evidence of past or present severe self-injury such as cauliflower ear, broken bones, extensive scarring, lacerations involving areas $>3 \times 3$ cm^2, autoamputation, loss of consciousness *and* one or more of the following: • signs of distress when inflicting injury such as crying • predilection for head as injury site	Opiate	Opiate antagonists, e.g. naltrexone
Repetitive and stereotypic	Autism	The topography of each movement is similar, not variable, as in hand-mouthing or repeated rubbing *and* two or more of the following are present: • short duration between movements (1–10 s) • tissue damage occurs only after repeated movements • co-occurring non-injurious stereotypies • diagnosis of autism or pervasive developmental disorder	Dopamine	Low dose of antipsychotics, e.g. haloperidol, risperidone
SIB with agitation when SIB interrupted	Obsessive compulsive behaviour	When SIB is interrupted, agitation or distress occurs such as crying, hyperventilation, aggression, pacing *and* one of more of the following is present: • mean rate of SIB is at least 100 incidents per hour • SIB stops during another activity but resumes within 30 s of its completion	Serotonin	SSRIs, e.g. fluoxetine, **or** tricyclic antidepressants, e.g. clomipramine

49

Table 5.2 *Continued*

Subtype	Key feature	Inclusion criteria	Neurotransmitter system	Treatment
Co-occurrence of SIB and agitation	High arousal	SIB is temporarily concurrent with agitation or aggression such as pacing, screaming, tachycardia *and* one of more of the following are present: • SIB rates vary by 50% or more per session • topographies consist of self-hitting • evidence of sleep or appetite disturbance	Noradrenaline	Anxiolytics, e.g. propranolol, **or** mood-stabilizing drugs, e.g. lithium
Multiple clinical features		The individual meets inclusion criteria of two or more of the other subtypes	Several of above	According to subtypes

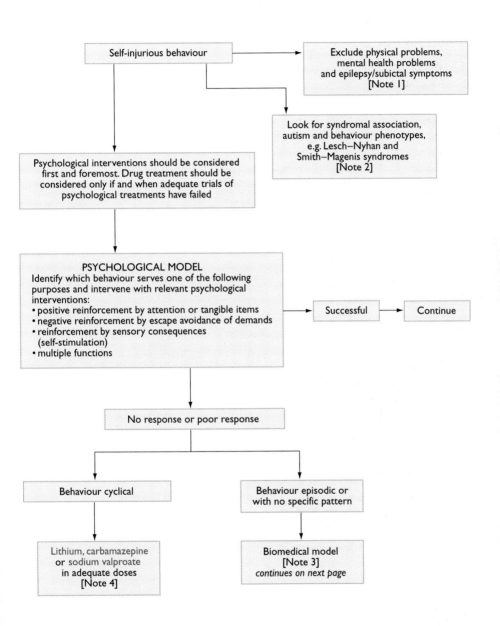

Algorithm 5.1   Treatment of self-injurious behaviour (SIB) in adults with LD

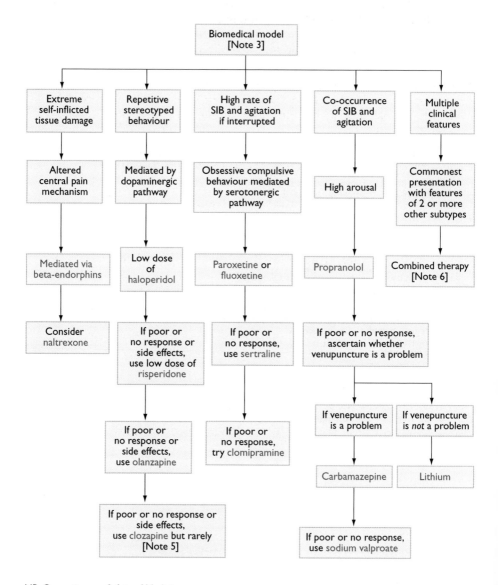

NB: Committee on Safety of Medicines
1. There is an increased risk of cerebrovascular adverse events in older
   patients with dementia treated with olanzapine or risperidone.
2. Please refer to caution regarding the use of SSRIs and SNRIs.

Figure 5.2 Treatment of self-injurious behaviour (SIB) in adults with LD *continued*

Note 1: *co-morbidity*. Individuals should be examined and treated for physical problems such as pain, infections, constipation and other medical conditions. Epilepsy, particularly that presenting as subclinical seizures, requires thorough investigation and treatment. Individuals should also be examined and treated for major mental disorders such as schizophrenia, delusional disorder, depressive disorder and bipolar mood disorder, and for other minor mental health problems.

Note 2: *syndromes*. For SIB in Lesch–Nyhan syndrome, a trial of naltrexone may first be considered. If this fails, one needs to consider a trial of olanzepine or clozapine. In Smith–Magenis syndrome, SIB has been found to respond to lithium and other mood-stabilizing drugs.

Note 3: *subtypes*. If treatment based on one subtype fails to elicit the desired response, an alternative subtype may be considered and the treatment changed accordingly.

Note 4: *mood-stabilizing drugs*. When one mood-stabilizing drug is found to be ineffective, another one may be considered.

Note 5: *clozapine*. SIB is not a licensed indication for the use of clozapine. Therefore, its use requires multidisciplinary agreement of the local trust and special permission by the Clozaril Monitoring Service.

Note 6: *combined therapy*. It is not advisable to combine more than two classes of drug. When prescribing more than two classes is unavoidable, a second opinion is advised. Possible combinations of more than one class of drug include:

- naltrexone and antipsychotic
- mood-stabilizer and antipsychotic
- mood-stabilizer and SSRI
- antipsychotic and SSRI (especially risperidone and paroxetine).

There is an increased risk of neurotoxicity when lithium is combined with carbamazepine.

Key references

Aman MG. Efficacy of psychotropic drugs for reducing self-injurious behaviour in the developmental disabilities. *Annals of Clinical Psychiatry* 1993; **5**: 177–188.

Amin P, Yeraghavi VK. Control of aggressive and self-mutilative behaviour in a mentally retarded patient with lithium. *Canadian Journal of Psychiatry* 1987; **32**: 162–163.

Buzan RD, Dubovsky SL, Treadway JT, Thomas M. Opiate antagonists for recurrent self-injurious behaviour in three mentally retarded adults. *Psychiatric Services* 1995; **46**: 511–512.

Casner JA, Weinheimer B, Gualtieri CT. Naltrexone and self-injurious behaviour: a retrospective population study. *Journal of Clinical Psychopharmacology* 1996; **16**: 389–394.

Clarke DJ. Psychopharmacology of severe self-injury associated with learning disabilities. *British Journal of Psychiatry* 1998; **172**: 3834–3894.

Favazza A, Rosenthal R. Diagnostic issues in self-mutilation. *Hospital and Community Psychiatry* 1993; **44**: 134–140.

Hassler F, Fsuch Asert JM. Psychopharmacological therapy of self-injurious behaviour in mentally retarded individuals. *Nervenarzt* 1999; **70**: 1025–1028.

Iwata BA, Dorsey MF, Stifer KJ, Bauman KE, Richman GS. Toward a functional analysis of self-injury. *Journal of Applied Behavioural Analysis* 1994; **27**: 197–209.

Lewis MH, Bodfish JW, Powell SB, Parker DE, Golden RN. Clomipramine treatment for self-injurious behaviour of individuals with mental retardation: a double-blind comparison with placebo. *American Journal of Mental Retardation* 1996; **100**: 654–665.

McDonough M, Hillery J, Kennedy N. Olanzapine for chronic, stereotypic self-injurious behaviour: a pilot study in seven adults with intellectual disability. *Journal of Intellectual Disability Research* 2000; **44**: 677–684.

Mace CF, Mauk JE. Biobehavioural diagnosis and treatment of self-injury. *Mental Retardation and Developmental Disabilities Research Reviews* 1995; **1**: 104–110.

Oliver C, Murphy GH, Corbett JA. Self-injurious behaviour in people with mental handicap: a total population study. *Journal of Mental Deficiency Research* 1987; **31**: 147–162.

Ricketts RW, Goza AB, Ellis CR, Singh YN, Singh NN, Cooke JC 3rd. Fluoxetine treatment of severe self-injury in young adults with mental retardation. *Journal of the American Academy of Child and Adolescent Psychiatry* 1993; **32**: 865–869.

Ruedrich S, Swales TP, Fossaceca C, Toliver J, Rutkowski A. Effect of divalproex sodium on aggression and self-injurious behaviour in adults with intellectual disability: a retrospective review. *Journal of Intellectual Disability Research* 1999; **43**: 105–111.

Schroeder SR. Dopaminergic mechanisms in self-injury. *Psychology in Mental Retardation and Developmental Disabilities* 1996; **22**: 10–13.

Wickham EA, Reed JV. Lithium for the control of aggressive and self-mutilating behaviour. *International Clinical Psychopharmacology* 1987; **2**: 181–190.

chapter 6

Aggression

Definition

Aggression is a severe form of behaviour involving damage to property and/or verbal and/or physical assault of another person. In the wider spectrum, aggression may be seen as part of challenging behaviour (CB). CB is defined as behaviour of such intensity, frequency or duration that the physical safety of the person or others is placed in serious jeopardy. Such behaviour may seriously limit or deny the individual access to the use of ordinary community facilities.

In addition to physical and verbal aggression, CB may include temper tantrums, unco-operativeness, attention-seeking behaviour, self-injury, hyperactivity, excessive noisiness, disturbing others at night, absconding, delinquency and/or sexual behaviour problems. Aggression that is chronic and persistent therefore poses serious problems for carers and professionals in providing adequate services for people with learning disability (LD).

Aggression has been studied extensively by behaviour-research scientists, psychologists, psychiatrists and others. Although aggression may be natural, some theories suggest that it may be acquired as a part of social learning. In the context of LD, frequent or chronic aggression is considered to be a pattern of maladaptive behaviour requiring evaluation and treatment.

Prevalence

People with LD are more susceptible to aggression than the general population. However, estimates of prevalence vary according to the definition of aggression, the sample population and the reliability of the methods of data collection. The prevalence ranges from 11% to 60%. Although physical and verbal aggression is generally the most frequently reported behaviour, many people also engage in the other forms of CB.

There are significant gender differences in both the presence and type of aggression. Proportionately more males than females engage in aggression, especially in physical aggression, destruction of property, temper tantrums and verbal abuse. Some studies have shown no difference.

Proportionately more individuals with moderate, severe and profound degrees of LD engage in acts of aggression than those with mild LD. For some individuals with no intelligible speech, aggression may serve as a form of communication. Unfortunately, over time, there is very little abatement in abnormal behaviour patterns in this group. While some studies have shown higher prevalence of aggression in younger age groups, others have found there is no association with age.

The prevalence of aggression is higher among people living in long-term institutions (35–38%) than among those in group homes (27%) or a community setting (9.7%).

Key points specific to learning disability

Factors affecting aggression

An understanding of the factors associated with aggression is essential for successful intervention. Individual characteristics such as age, sex and degree of LD, and factors relating to the situation and the environment should be considered. In recent years, there has been a move toward person–situation models with inclusion of environmental factors.

Applied behaviour analysis or functional analysis

This type of analysis is mandatory when considering aggression in people with LD. The functional relationship between environmental conditions and CB requires detailed exploration.

Functional analysis is often limited to the relationship between the behaviour and the immediate environment (antecedents and consequences of the behaviour). Such a narrow concept, however, risks missing important information, which includes personal attributes (coping and communication skills) and factors in the wider environment (available social support). People with LD change their roles and tasks over their life span. The demands of such changes may have an effect on personal and environmental variables, resulting in improvement or worsening of the aggression.

Physical or psychiatric illness

Physical or psychiatric illness often precipitates aggression in individuals with LD. Physical pain such as that of recurrent otitis media or dysmenorrhoea may frustrate an individual with LD who lacks the verbal skills to communicate specific details about the distress. The doctor should carry out a medical examination for a physical cause of the aggression, especially in those who have minimal communication skills. Individuals who have mania or paranoid schizophrenic illnesses are often hostile. Others, including those with pervasive developmental disorders, often react aggressively when their territorial space is invaded or their routine is upset. Confusional states and drug misuse are rare causes of aggression in people with LD.

Any physical or psychiatric illness needs to be treated separately from aggression.

Aggression and epilepsy

Aggression in people who have both LD and epilepsy is not uncommon, although its aetiology may not be clear. Having established the presence of active epilepsy, it is important to determine whether the aggression is peri-ictal (occurs immediately before, during or immediately after the seizure) or occurs between seizures. The ideal way of linking aggression with peri-ictal phenomena is by ambulatory electroencephalogram (EEG) monitoring.

Maladaptive behaviours and dementia

People with dementia in the general population often show maladaptive behaviour. Studies have shown similar findings in those with LD who develop dementia. Common features are agitation, irritability, aggression and lack of a sense of danger.

Individuals with Down syndrome who develop dementia are more likely to have characteristics of maladaptive behaviour, such as disturbed sleep, restlessness, hyperactivity or aggression, than others in the LD population with dementia.

Treatment

Drug treatment of aggression in the absence of functional psychiatric illness may be considered as a last resort and should be undertaken only along with other non-pharmacological approaches including psychological therapies. Input from other professionals, including speech and language therapists and behaviour therapists, is essential, especially if the cause of aggression is suspected to be that of maladaptive learning, environmental problems or communication difficulties. The choice of drug treatment of chronic aggression depends on the type of aggression, the degree of sympathetic arousal, the extent of hyperactivity and the presence of epilepsy or an abnormal EEG.

If aggression is related to seizures (peri-ictal), the behaviour tends to respond to adequate seizure control through the use of appropriate antiepileptic drugs. People with interictal aggression should be treated in a similar way to those without epilepsy. Treatment with most psychotropic medications, including antipsychotics and antidepressants, lowers the seizure threshold. This is an important consideration when selecting the dose of medication.

Where there is evidence of recent or past mood disturbance or if there is a periodic cycle of aggression, treatment should be with lithium or other mood stabilizers. In the absence of a clear affective component, lithium is more effective than other mood stabilizers. Carbamazepine or sodium valproate is generally used when there is a history of epilepsy or an abnormal EEG.

Beta-blockers, such as propranolol, may be tried if there are features of autonomic hyperarousal or associated somatic features of anxiety.

Antidepressant drugs, especially selective serotonin re-uptake inhibitors (SSRIs), have been used to control impulsive behaviour in those with normal intelligence. It has been postulated that these drugs will also reduce impulsive aggression in those with LD, although the evidence for this is limited.

In practice, people with LD who have a history of aggression are most commonly treated with antipsychotics. The typical antipsychotics have several disadvantages, including tardive dyskinesia after long-term use and withdrawal symptoms after sudden cessation of treatment (nausea, anorexia, restlessness and painful muscles). These may contribute to aggression in those who cannot communicate effectively. People with LD are susceptible to movement disorders due to the underlying neurological damage.

In spite of the extensive use of antipsychotics to control aggressive or maladaptive behaviour in adults with LD, the evidence of the effectiveness of the drugs remains weak. A systematic review of randomized, controlled trials suggested that the effectiveness of antipsychotics in this situation is not proven. It is advisable to identify the target symptoms, record baseline parameters, monitor their efficacy and note any adverse effects. Antipsychotics should be used with caution until further information is available.

The Maudsley Guidelines should be followed for guidance on rapid tranquillization. It is important to note the following:

- Chlorpromazine is *no longer* recommended because of concerns about hypotension and tachycardia.

- Intramuscular diazepam is *not* recommended because of irregular absorption and long half-life.

- The National Institute for Clinical Excellence (NICE) recommends intramuscular olanzapine.

Algorithm 6.1 should be used as a guide only for treatment of adults with both LD and aggression.

Note 1: *delirium.* Common causes of delirium are infections, trauma, postictal state, hepatic or renal disease, metabolic disorders, fluid or electrolyte imbalances, intoxication or withdrawal of substances, thiamine deficiency and encephalopathy.

Note 2: *rapid tranquillization.* Each mental health trust has its own policy for the administration of rapid tranquillization. In addition, NICE has published guidance for the control of an acute psychotic episode.

Note 3: *concurrent prescription of psychotropic medication.* The concurrent use of two or more classes of psychotropic drugs should be avoided whenever possible. If two psychotropic drugs need to be prescribed, the rationale should be clearly stated and documented in the patient's medical notes. The patient should be monitored regularly for the side effects of each drug and any drug interactions. It is advisable to seek a second opinion when more than two classes of psychotropic drugs are thought to be necessary.

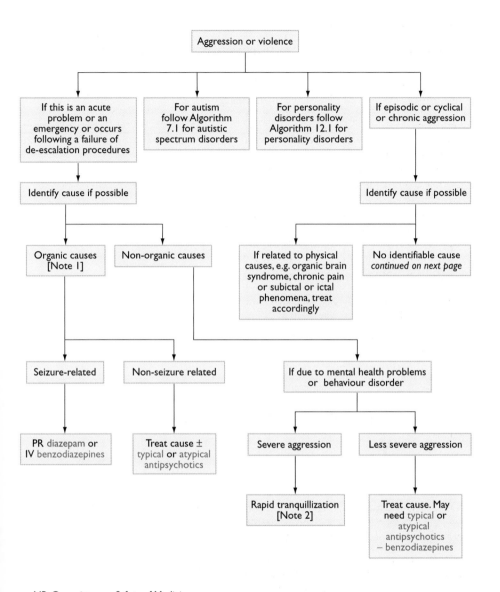

No identifiable cause
continued on next page

NB: Committee on Safety of Medicines
1. There is an increased risk of cerebrovascular adverse events in older
   patients with dementia treated with olanzapine or risperidone.
2. Please refer to caution regarding the use of SSRIs and SNRIs.

Figure 6.1   Treatment of aggression in adults with LD

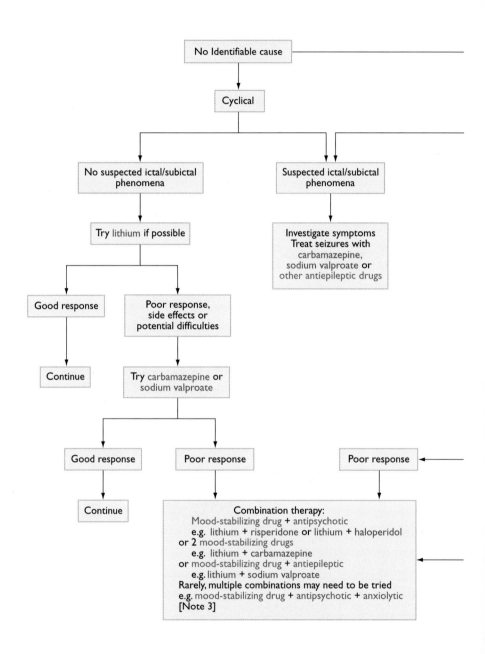

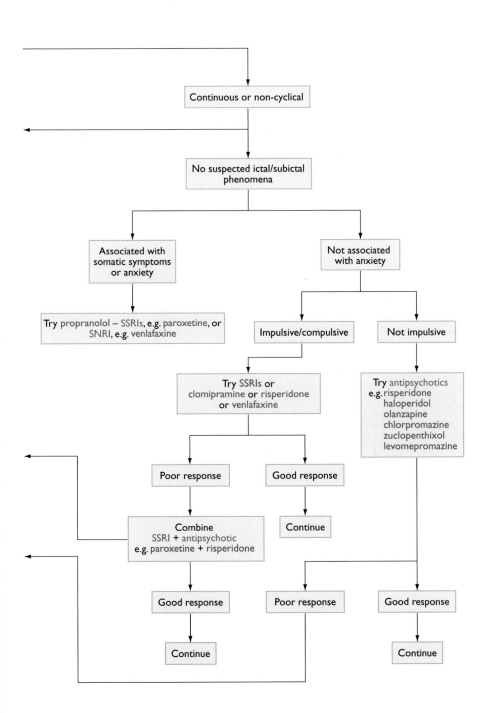

Key references

Branford D, Bhaumik S, Naik B. Selective serotonin re-uptake inhibitors for the treatment of perseverative and maladaptive behaviours of people with intellectual disability. *Journal of Intellectual Disability Research* 1998; **42**: 301–306.

Brylewski J, Duggan L. Antipsychotic medication for challenging behaviour in people with intellectual disability: a systematic review of randomised controlled trials. *Journal of Intellectual Disability Research* 1999; **43**: 360–371.

Cohen SA, Ihrig K, Lotts RS, Kerrick JM. Risperidone for aggression and self-injurious behaviour in adults with mental retardation. *Journal of Autism and Developmental Disorders* 1998; **28**: 229–233.

Cooper S-A. A population-based health survey of maladaptive behaviours associated with dementia in elderly people with learning disabilities. *Journal of Intellectual Disability Research* 1997; **41**: 481–487.

Harris P. The nature and extent of aggression amongst people with learning difficulties (mental handicap) in a single health district. *Journal of Intellectual Disability Research* 1993; **37**: 221–242.

Haspel T. Beta-blockers and the treatment of aggression. *Harvard Review of Psychiatry* 1995; **2**: 274–281.

Langee HR. A retrospective study of mentally retarded patients with behavioural disorders who were treated with carbamazepine. *American Journal of Mental Retardation* 1989; **93**: 640–643.

Lindenmayer JP, Kotsaftis A. Use of sodium valproate in violent and aggressive behaviors: a critical review. *Journal of Clinical Psychiatry* 2000; **61**: 123–128.

Reid AH, Ballinger BR. Behaviour symptoms among severely and profoundly mentally retarded patients: a 16–18 year follow-up study. *British Journal of Psychiatry* 1995; **167**: 452–455.

Sigafoos J, Elkins J, Kerr M, Attwood T. A survey of aggression among a population of persons with intellectual disability in Queensland. *Journal of Intellectual Disability Research* 1994; **38**: 369–381.

Smith S, Branford D, Collacott RA, Cooper SA, McGrother C. Prevalence and cluster typology of maladaptive behaviour in a geographically defined population of adults with learning disabilities. *British Journal of Psychiatry* 1996; **169**: 219–227.

Wickham EA, Reed JV. Lithium for the control of aggressive and self-mutilating behaviour. *International Clinical Psychopharmacology* 1987; **2**: 181–190.

chapter 7

Autistic spectrum disorders

Definition

Autism or autistic spectrum disorders (ASD) comprise a spectrum of severe developmental and neuropsychiatric disorders that are usually apparent by the age of 3 years. Kanner gave the first detailed description of autism in his paper 'Autistic disturbances of affective contact' in 1943. From her field research, Wing later drew up a triad of behavioural criteria for the diagnosis of autistic disorder, as shown in the box.

Wing's triad of impairments for autistic disorder

- qualitative impairment in reciprocal social interaction
- qualitative impairment in verbal and non-verbal communication and in imaginative activity
- a markedly restricted repertoire of activities and interests.

These impairments are found in people with ASD throughout the range of intelligence and in all the clinical subtypes. Characteristic sensory and motor abnormalities are also commonly described (Table 7.1).

Prevalence

ASD are considerably more common than was previously believed. Studies have shown that the prevalence is between 7 and 17 per 10 000 children of all ages, and between 12 and 20 per 10 000 children of school age.

Table 7.1 Characteristics of autistic spectrum disorders

Characteristics	Key features
Social impairment	• Variable in degree and nature • Difficulty with social cues affecting reciprocal social interaction, joint interactive play and joint attention behaviour • Failure to recognize emotional cues, resulting in inappropriate responses to distress in others, reflecting a wider lack of empathy
Language abnormalities	• Both verbal and non-verbal spheres of language are affected • Expressive function is more affected that receptive language • Both symbolic and pragmatic language abnormalities occur, including echolalia, abnormal prosody, pronoun reversal and lack of variation in the quality of speech
Limited imagination	• Interests and activities are limited to a few circumscribed themes, with a lack of spontaneity, imaginativeness and creativity • Activities are typically repetitive and stereotyped, with interest being shown in a part of an object rather than in the whole • There may be compulsive routines and unusual attachments, often resulting in a large collection and storage problems • Any unexpected change may result in great distress to the autistic person, who may become very agitated and aggressive
Sensory-motor abnormalities	• Abnormal perceptions, especially hearing and vision, may result in stimulus overload • A lack of internal monitoring of time and space may make the person unable to think in a sequential framework • Motor dysfunction (stereotypies) may present as hand-flapping or bouncing up and down and/or gyration, which become marked when the person is excited or distressed

ASD are also more common in people with learning disability (LD) than in the general population, with a prevalence of 5% in those with mild LD and 15% in those with moderate or severe LD. Of those with the condition, 75–90% have LD. All studies report an excess of boys with ASD, and most give a male:female ratio of between 3:1 and 4:1. Among those with the condition and a severe to profound degree of LD, the male:female ratio approaches 1:1. There is a relatively low prevalence of girls with ASD in the higher intelligence ranges. This suggests a sex-linked genetic mechanism.

Aetiology

Autistic traits are recognized more often than a clear-cut diagnosis of ASD. One study showed that 40% of adults with LD have autistic traits. The pathogenesis of ASD is not clearly established. The proposed hypotheses range from psychological to neurobiological theories. The recent evidence favours a neurobiological explanation.

Psychological theories

There has been much debate about whether ASD are primarily an interpersonal impairment, a cognitive defect or a failure in the development of language, communication and social skills.

Theory of mind hypothesis

Theory of mind refers to the ability of normal children to attribute mental states such as beliefs, desires and intentions to themselves and other people as a way of making sense of and predicting behaviour. It has been suggested that the impairments seen in autistic children arise because they lack a theory of mind.

Central coherence theory

Recent work has suggested that there may be more fundamental deficits in ASD such as an inability to visualize relationships between objects or to extract meaning from piecemeal information.

Neurobiological theories

Computed tomography (CT) and magnetic resonance imaging (MRI) studies

The following structural abnormalities have been reported on CT scans of individuals with ASD:

- reversed cerebral asymmetries
- enlargement of the lateral and third ventricles
- decreased radiodensity of the caudate nuclei.

However, there have been problems in reproducing these results and in finding a consistent pattern.

A recent MRI study found developmental cortical malformations and delayed maturation of the frontal lobes in people with ASD. It has been suggested that abnormal neuronal migration occurring perhaps in the first 6 months of gestation accounts for the cerebral cortical defects and hypoplasia. The underlying cause of the failed cell migration remains unknown, but viral and immunological factors need to be considered.

Neurochemical findings

Abnormalities have been found in monoamine chemistry, peptides, amino acids and neuroendocrine functioning:

- Raised platelet serotonin (5-hydroxytryptamine or 5-HT) levels are consistently raised in 30% of autistic people. Similar levels are found in their first-degree relatives.

- Levels of serotomin in autistic people with affected siblings are significantly higher than in autistic people without affected siblings, and the levels in both groups are higher than in controls.

- The dopamine system may also be abnormal, with low levels of dopa-hydroxylase found in probands and first-degree relatives compared with controls.

- Raised urinary and cerebrospinal fluid levels of homovanillic acid and elevated plasma noradrenaline have been reported in people with ASD.

- Raised whole-blood serotonin levels have been found in specific subgroups of people with ASD, including those with fragile X syndrome.

- Growing evidence of abnormalities of the hypothalamic–pituitary axis suggests that abnormalities of the monoamine oxidase and indoleamine systems may be involved in ASD.

Disturbance in any of these systems could greatly interfere with normal cognitive processes. Perceptual pathways are all mediated by neurotransmitters and homeostatic neuroregulators. However, the specific defects that explain Wing's triad remains elusive.

Genetic influences

There is now growing evidence that genetic factors play an important role in ASD:

- The frequency of ASD in siblings of autistic children is 50 times higher than in the general population. About 15% of siblings of people with ASD have lesser developmental disorders of speech, language or reading skills. It is suggested that it is these psychological characteristics, rather than a global cognitive defect, that are inherited.

- Same-sex twin studies in ASD have shown that monozygotic concordance rates (36–89%) are much higher than dizygotic concordance rates (0%). Most of the non-autistic co-twins had some form of cognitive impairment, usually a speech or language impairment. The monozygotic concordance rates for these lesser impairments (82%) were higher than dizygotic concordance rates (10%).

- Parents of autistic individuals have higher ratings than parents of controls on a standardized personality interview for the characteristics of being aloof, tactless, undemonstrative and unresponsive.

Evidence from the family and twin studies taken together suggests that the ASD phenotype extends beyond autism as it is traditionally diagnosed. The condition is likely to be heterogeneous and may involve several genes.

Associated medical conditions

One in four children with ASD has an associated medical condition (Table 7.2). It is possible that these conditions may have a common underlying genetic aetiology, ASD being caused through a final common pathway.

Table 7.2 Medical conditions associated with autistic spectrum disorders

Classification of conditions	Examples
Chromosome abnormalities	Fragile X syndrome, Rett syndrome, Williams syndrome
Neurocutaneous disorders	Tuberous sclerosis
Metabolic diseases	Mucopolysaccharidosis, phenylketonuria
Infections	Encephalitis, cytomegalovirus infection, maternal rubella

Key points specific to learning disability

There appears to be no cure for ASD. The clinical focus is on the management of maladaptive behaviours and functioning rather than on the primary condition. Management approaches include psychological education, family support, behaviour therapy, environmental manipulation and special education. In addition to these therapeutic approaches, drug treatment of maladaptive behaviours may be necessary in certain circumstances.

Stereotyped behaviour (rituals)

Stereotypic and ritualistic activities interfere with learning and are thus disruptive. They include the development of fixed routines. When these are interrupted, they may cause great distress, resulting in disturbed behaviour. The rituals in ASD are not accompanied by obsessional thoughts and may be comforting (unlike the compulsions seen in obsessive compulsive disorder).

The management of the rituals in ASD differs from the conventional treatment of those in obsessive compulsive disorder. However, serotonin selective re-uptake inhibitors (SSRIs) may be useful in treating repetitive behaviours.

Autistic spectrum disorders and aggressive behaviour

Aggression occurs frequently. It may represent a means of communication, particularly in response to a perceived threat or in those with limited verbal abilities, to gain attention, express distress or relieve boredom. Any strategy should be based on functional analysis of the behaviour, with contingency management being the primary objective of the intervention. Drugs may be used as a last resort to control aggressive behaviour.

Autistic spectrum disorders and self-injurious behaviour

The neurotransmitter hypotheses in the biomedical model of self-injurious behaviour (Table 5.2) may explain the underlying aetiology of self-injurious behaviour in people with ASD. However, before concentrating on biological models, it is useful to identify the antecedents of self-injurious behaviour (change in routine, social cues or the environment), and to note whether the behaviour is being used as a form of communication.

Autistic spectrum disorders and epilepsy

There is an increased incidence of epilepsy and abnormal electroencephalogram (EEG) findings in people with ASD. There is an initial increase in the incidence of epilepsy during early childhood and a later increase during adolescence. The incidence rises to 25–40% by early adulthood. Generalized seizures are the most common form of epilepsy. Complex partial seizures may be more frequent than previously estimated.

The onset of seizures in adolescence is sometimes, but not usually, associated with marked behaviour changes and aggression. EEG abnormalities have been estimated to occur in 10–83% of people with ASD. Around 58% show abnormalities on repeat EEGs. The most common findings are diffuse or focal spikes, slow waves, and paroxysmal spike and wave activity with a mixed discharge. Most abnormalities are bilateral. Unilateral findings tend not to be clearly localized.

Autistic spectrum disorders and attention deficit hyperactivity disorder

A large number of people with ASD show significant levels of inattention, impulsivity and hyperactivity. These behaviours are typically associated with attention deficit hyperactivity disorder. Stimulants are beneficial in some people. However, adverse effects, such as social withdrawal, irritability and loss of appetite, may be marked at higher doses.

Treatment

Figure 7.1 should be used as a guide only for the treatment of adults with both LD and ASD.

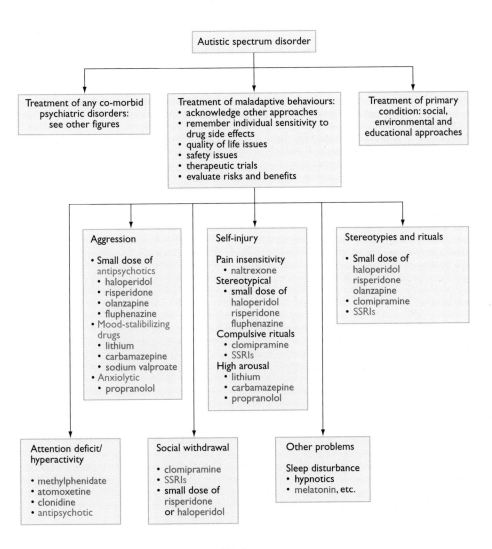

Autistic spectrum disorder

Treatment of any co-morbid psychiatric disorders: see other figures

Treatment of maladaptive behaviours:
• acknowledge other approaches
• remember individual sensitivity to drug side effects
• quality of life issues
• safety issues
• therapeutic trials
• evaluate risks and benefits

Treatment of primary condition: social, environmental and educational approaches

Aggression
• Small dose of antipsychotics
  • haloperidol
  • risperidone
  • olanzapine
  • fluphenazine
• Mood-stalibilizing drugs
  • lithium
  • carbamazepine
  • sodium valproate
• Anxiolytic
  • propranolol

Self-injury
Pain insensitivity
  • naltrexone
Stereotypical
  • small dose of haloperidol risperidone fluphenazine
Compulsive rituals
  • clomipramine
  • SSRIs
High arousal
  • lithium
  • carbamazepine
  • propranolol

Stereotypies and rituals
• Small dose of haloperidol risperidone olanzapine
  • clomipramine
  • SSRIs

Attention deficit/ hyperactivity
• methylphenidate
• atomoxetine
• clonidine
• antipsychotic

Social withdrawal
  • clomipramine
  • SSRIs
  • small dose of risperidone or haloperidol

Other problems
Sleep disturbance
  • hypnotics
  • melatonin, etc.

NB: Committee on Safety of Medicines
1. There is an increased risk of cerebrovascular adverse events in older patients with dementia treated with olanzapine or risperidone.
2. Please refer to caution regarding the use of SSRIs and SNRIs.

Algorithm 7.1 Treatment of autistic spectrum disorder in adults with LD

Key references

Baron-Cohen S. *Mind Blindness. An Essay on Autism and Theory of Mind.* Cambridge, MA: MIT Press, 1951.

Bhaumik S, Branford D, McGrother C, Thorp C. Autistic traits in adults with learning disabilities. *British Journal of Psychiatry* 1997; **170**: 502–506.

Frith U. *Autism: Explaining the Enigma.* Oxford: Blackwell, 1989.

Kanner L. Autistic disturbances of affective contact. *Nervous Child* 1943; **2**: 217–250.

Nordin V, Gillbert G. Autistic spectrum disorders in children with physical or mental disability or both. I. Clinical and epidemiological aspects. *Developmental Medicine and Child Neurology* 1996; **38**: 297–313.

Steffenburg S, Gillberg C. Autism and autistic-like conditions in Swedish rural and urban areas: a population study. *British Journal of Psychiatry* 1986; **149**: 81–87.

Wing L, Gould J. Severe impairments of social interaction and associated abnormalities in children: epidemiology and classification. *Journal of Autism and Developmental Disorders* 1979; **9**: 11–19.

chapter 8

Attention deficit hyperactivity disorder

Definition

The cardinal features of attention deficit hyperactivity disorder (ADHD) are extreme and persistent restlessness, sustained and prolonged motor overactivity, and difficulty in maintaining attention. These behaviours begin in childhood and are relatively chronic. They are not explained by gross neurological, sensory, language or motor impairment or by learning disabilities or severe emotional disturbance. These difficulties are typically associated with deficits in rule-governed behaviour or in maintaining a consistent pattern of work performance over time. Rule-governed behaviour refers to the capacity for language such as commands, directions, instructions or descriptions to direct an individual's course of action.

The DSM-IV and the ICD-10 are the main two systems of diagnostic criteria. The recent editions of these have brought the definitions of ADHD and hyperkinetic disorder (HD) closer together (Table 8.1).

Estimates of the prevalence of ADHD vary according to the diagnostic criteria and the terminology used. In a review of six international epidemiological studies using DSM-IV criteria, the prevalence of ADHD in children ranged from 2.0% to 6.3%. A Canadian study found a lower prevalence in adolescence: 1.4% in boys and 1.0% in girls. Using ICD-10 criteria, a study of pre-schoolboys in the UK found that the prevalence was 1.7%. The disorder is more common in boys and in lower socioeconomic settings. ADHD is diagnosed more frequently in the USA than in the UK.

Prevalence

About 10–20% of children with learning disability (LD) have ADHD-like symptoms such as inattention, hyperactivity and impulsivity.

Table 8.1 Diagnostic criteria for attention deficit hyperactivity disorder in adults

	DSM-IV *Attention deficit hyperactivity disorder*	ICD-10 *Hyperkinetic disorder*
Diagnostic criteria		
Age of onset	Before the age of 7 years	Before the age of 6 years
Cardinal features	*Either* inattention *or* hyperactivity	*Both* inattention *and* hyperactivity
Presence of	**≥6 inattentive symptoms**, e.g. ● has difficulty in sustaining attention ● fails to give close attention to details ● does not seem to be listening when spoken to directly ● does not follow through on instructions ● has difficulty organizing tasks/activities ● is easily distracted by outside stimuli ● is often forgetful in daily activities **and/or** **≥6 hyperactive-impulsive symptoms**, e.g. ● fidgets with hands or feet ● cannot remain seated ● excessive running about or climbing ● has difficulty engaging in quiet activities ● always 'on the go'; 'driven by a motor' ● often talks incessantly	**≥6 inattentive symptoms**, e.g. ● poor attention ● prematurely breaks off from tasks ● leaves activities unfinished ● loses interest in one task when diverted to another ● flitting and fleeing activity ● lack of sustained purposeful action **and** **≥3 hyperactive symptoms**, e.g. ● marked motor overactivity ● inability to keep still ● excessive restlessness ● excessive noisiness or talkativeness **and** **1 impulsive symptom**, e.g. ● acts impatiently and impulsively ● acts without due care and attention
Subtypes	● Predominantly inattentive ● Predominantly hyperactive-impulsive ● Combined	● Disturbance of activity and attention ● Hyperkinetic conduct disorder

Table 8.1 *Continued*

	DSM-IV *Attention deficit hyperactivity disorder*	ICD-10 *Hyperkinetic disorder*
Cross-situational pervasiveness	There needs to be evidence that the above criteria are *fully met* in one situation, and that impairment is *present* in a second (no stipulation of the number and severity of the symptoms in the latter)	All the above criteria must be *fully met both* at home *and* in other situations (e.g. classroom, clinic)
Co-morbidity	Commonly coexists with • pervasive developmental disorders • other major psychiatric disorders	

Several retrospective and prospective studies have indicated that between 30% and 70% of children with ADHD continue to have some symptoms into early adulthood. They may become less impulsive and hyperactive but remain more distractible, restless, emotionally immature and aggressive than other adults. When compared with the general population, those with ADHD have a higher risk of affective disorders, substance abuse and personality disorders (mainly antisocial and sometimes borderline). Symptoms of inattentiveness and impulsiveness occur across a range of psychological and medical disorders such as depression, anxiety, personality disorders, head injuries and chronic substance abuse.

Aetiology

Genetic factors

A genetic basis for ADHD is suggested by a study of adopted children and by comparisons of monozygotic and dizygotic twins. Probands with ADHD had more first-degree relatives with ADHD or with antisocial and major depressive disorders than controls. A model postulating a single major gene defect remains to be confirmed.

Neurobiological factors

Brain imaging studies

SPECT scans (single-photon emission computed tomography) of individuals with ADHD have shown decreases in cerebral blood flow in the striatal region, which increases after treatment with methylphenidate.

PET (positron emission tomography) scans in adults with ADHD have shown decreased global glucose metabolism, primarily in the prefrontal and premotor cortex compared with control subjects without ADHD.

Neurochemical studies

No single brain region or neurotransmitter dysfunction adequately explains the clinical presentation of ADHD. The condition probably involves interaction of several neurotransmitters in different regions of the brain.

Dopamine hypothesis

- Selective brain dopamine depletion in developing rats resulted in hyperactivity when the animals reached maturity.

- Investigations of cerebrospinal fluid and monoamine metabolites in children with ADHD showed altered levels of brain dopamine.

- Methylphenidate has been shown to activate dopamine neurons by decreasing the re-uptake of dopamine through dopamine transporters.

- Stimulants have been shown to possess dopamine-releasing effects.

Noradrenaline hypothesis

- Defective inhibition of the noradrenergic locus caeruleus leads to a state of hypervigilance and ADHD-like symptoms.

- Clonidine acts by direct stimulation of presynaptic α_2-adrenergic sites that inhibit the release of noradrenaline, leading to an increase in postsynaptic noradrenergic sensitivity.

- Atomoxetine is a selective noradrenaline re-uptake inhibitor.

- Antidepressants, such as desipramine, may involve a noradrenergic mechanism of action. They show modest effectiveness in ADHD.

Serotonin hypothesis

- Serotonin (5-hydroxytryptamine or 5-HT) is more effective in treating concurrent mood disorder than in ADHD alone.

- No clear pattern of change in platelet and blood serotonin has been shown in people with ADHD.

Social cognitive domain

- Failure to activate somatic (body) states deprives an individual of an automatic device to signal the harmful consequences of decisions. Awareness of past choices and the results of such choices are essential for modifying behaviours.

- There is difficulty in linking affect to cognition, and deficient automatic response to social stimuli.

- People with ADHD show deficits in internal planning, organizing and online monitoring, as assessed through a story-retelling task.

Executive dysfunction syndrome

This is characterized by difficulties in planning and sequencing complex behaviours, difficulties in paying attention to several components of a problem at any one time, difficulties in inhibiting inappropriate response tendencies, difficulties in resisting distraction and interference and difficulties in sustaining a behaviour for a relatively long period of time.

Many studies using neuropsychological tests suggest that the frontal lobes are involved in regulating attention, especially the prefrontal system.

Key points specific to learning disability

Hyperkinetic syndrome and brain damage

Children with evidence of brain damage, such as those with epilepsy or cerebral palsy, have high rates of hyperkinetic syndrome. Rates are higher in children with LD, especially if this is severe, with around 10% of individuals being affected overall. Hyperactivity, inattention and impulsiveness are evident at school, at home and in social situations. The extent of these behaviours depends on the demands being made on the child and on the external controls and reinforcers.

ADHD and genetic disorder

ADHD has been found to be associated with a number of genetic disorders, including fragile X syndrome, tuberous sclerosis and Smith–Magenis syndrome.

ADHD and epilepsy

A number of children with atypical and intractable forms of epilepsy have behaviour problems and are hyperactive. Improvement in seizure control or change in antiepileptic treatment does not necessarily reduce this behaviour.

ADHD and other disorders

ADHD is reported in approximately one-third of people who have Gilles de la Tourette syndrome. The symptoms of ADHD may fluctuate, as motor and vocal tics do. A high level of activity and short attention span may also be secondary features of autism. These often respond favourably to stimulants.

Treatment

Current issues in the treatment of children with ADHD

The National Institute for Clinical Excellence (NICE) guidelines for the treatment of children with ADHD should be considered, because adults with LD and ADHD are treated on similar principles.

The use of stimulants in children with ADHD is controversial. The primary concerns are adverse reactions, compliance, fluctuating plasma drug levels (with immediate release preparations) and the possibility of drug misuse. Despite these concerns, stimulants have an essential role to play in the management of ADHD.

The MTA study (National Institute for Mental Health Collaborative Multisite Multimodal Treatment Study of Children with Attention Deficit/Hyperactivity Disorder, USA—MTA Co-operative Group 1999) attempted to address these issues by measuring outcomes across a wide range of domains, using 19 different measures. The secondary analyses have been used to develop rational prescribing of stimulants. The outcomes from the MTA study have been used in the NICE guidelines for the treatment of ADHD.

Treatment of ADHD in adults without LD

Stimulants are useful in the treatment of ADHD, especially if disruptive behaviours are present. These behaviours include restlessness, hyperactivity, off-task behaviour, aggression, talking out of turn, out-of-seat behaviour, irritability, inability to follow directions, poor cooperation, opposition and non-compliance with rules. Stimulants have been shown to be the most efficacious of all drugs studied in improving symptoms of ADHD. Double-blind, controlled studies and case studies have consistently reflected the benefits of stimulants for symptoms of ADHD.

Methylphenidate has been the most widely studied stimulant, and it is the most popular. The majority of studies in adults show that approximately two-thirds of adults with ADHD have a good response to the drug. Several doses of methylphenidate have been recommended, ranging from 20 to 90 mg/day. The most common regime for methylphenidate is a total of 40 mg/day in divided doses.

The important side effects of methylphenidate in adults are as follows:

- decreased appetite—at a high dose

- insomnia—no significant dose-related effect

- headache—no dose-response effect

- stomach pain—dose-response effect.

Other side effects include sadness and a tendency to cry, anxiety, irritability, euphoria, nail-biting, talkativeness, nightmares, tics and nervous movements, dizziness, drowsiness and staring. In children, there is a significant risk of growth retardation with methylphenidate therapy, and monitoring of weight and scheduling of drug holidays are important. In all age groups, hallucinations and psychoses are rare but may be severe; they tend to occur with the first dose or when the dose is increased.

Dexamfetamine has a stimulant action similar to that of methylphenidate. It is beneficial in the treatment of adult ADHD in doses of up to 30 mg/day.

Antidepressants have been shown to be effective in reducing symptoms of ADHD in adults. If an individual has difficulty in sleeping or is restless as the result of treatment with a stimulant, an antidepressant may be the treatment of choice. Antidepressants may also help to alleviate symptoms of anxiety in adults with co-morbid ADHD. In general, lower doses are suggested for the treatment of ADHD than for depression:

- imipramine 10–20 mg/day (to a maximum dose of 200 mg/day in adults)

- nortriptyline 10 mg/day (to a maximum dose of 150 mg/day in adults; plasma nortriptyline levels should be monitored in doses above 100 mg/day)

- fluoxetine 20 mg/day.

Clonidine has been shown to be effective in some individuals with ADHD, especially those with aggression and tic disorders. The main side effect is sedation.

Atomoxetine is a specific noradrenaline re-uptake inhibitor that has been shown to have comparable efficacy to methylphenidate. There is no indication that atomexetine adversely affects epilepsy or tics, or has misuse potential. It is licensed for the treatment of both adults and children with ADHD. For individuals weighing less than 70 kg, the dose is based on weight. The approximate starting dose is 0.5 mg/kg per day for a minimum of 7 days, and the recommended maintenance dose is 1.2 mg/kg per day. For individuals weighing 70 kg or over, the starting dose is 40 mg/day, and the recommended maintenance dose is 80 mg/day.

Several new non-stimulant drugs are undergoing clinical trials and are likely to be available in the near future. Nicotine patches and ABT-418, a nicotinic agonist acting on the central nervous system, have also shown positive results in open trials.

Treatment of ADHD in adults with learning disability

Drugs provide effective treatment for ADHD in adults. The severity of symptoms, co-morbid disorders and the effectiveness of non-pharmaceutical interventions need to be considered before starting drug treatment.

People with LD are treated less frequently with stimulants than the general population. This may be due to LD's being an exclusion criterion in clinical trials. Initial surveys showed that 3.4% of adults with LD living in the community and 2–3% of those living in institutions were taking stimulants.

There appears to be a relationship between the level of cognitive ability and the effectiveness of stimulants. Reviews suggest that the early studies focused on people with severe and profound LD who had a variety of behavioural difficulties, including hyperactivity. The majority of these studies did not show any statistically significant improvement in behaviour. However, studies that included people with mild and moderate LD who had clear symptoms of ADHD showed the beneficial effect of stimulants on behaviour. Case selection appears to be a major determinant of effectiveness. Carefully selected people with severe or profound LD may respond to a stimulant alone or in combination with other medications such as clonidine.

Several mechanisms have been suggested for this differential response to stimulants. One theory suggests that stimulants may increase the focus of attention. The attention span of people with ADHD and severe LD may show little improvement because their attention is overfocused. Another theory suggests that an intact frontal lobe system is necessary for an adequate response. Cortical hypoplasia, a frequent neuropathological finding in people with LD, may be a factor in the poor response to stimulants. However, these hypotheses are speculative. The mechanism of attention deficit may be quite different from that of hyperactivity.

All the drugs previously discussed for the symptomatic treatment of ADHD in adults without LD may be used in adults with LD. The side effects of stimulants in people with both ADHD and LD are similar to those for adults in the general population with ADHD. Antipsychotic medication, such as low doses of haloperidol, may also be used to control disruptive behaviour, including aggression and hyperactivity. However, more recent atypical antipsychotics, such as risperidone, should be considered before typical antipsychotics, as they are less likely to cause extrapyramidal symptoms, tardive dyskinesia and other serious side effects.

Figure 8.1 should be used as a guide only for the treatment of adults with both LD and ADHD.

Note 1: *methylphenidate*. Methylphenidate should be used only in patients without tics. It should be used with caution in patients with a history of epilepsy and in those who are underweight. If a patient has sleep disturbance, a diagnosis of mania or psychosis should be excluded before starting treatment. If weight loss or difficulty with getting off to sleep becomes a problem when using a sustained-release preparation, this should be replaced by an immediate-release preparation and the timing of administration adjusted accordingly.

Note 2: *clonidine*. When using clonidine, it is important to monitor blood pressure, and to look for signs and symptoms of depression and unexplained abdominal pain.

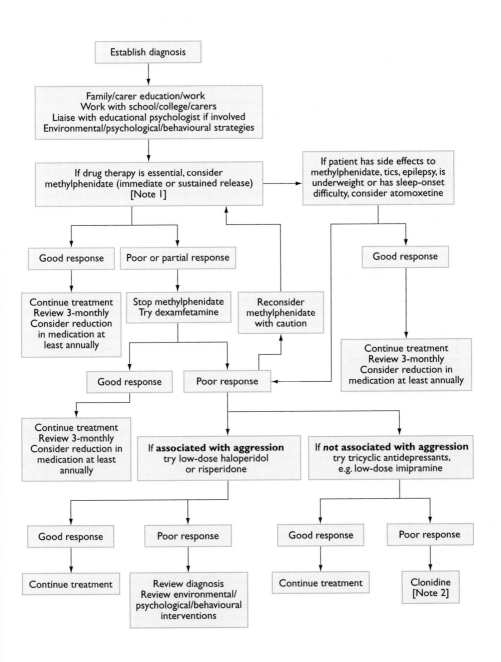

Algorithm 8.1 Drug treatment of attention deficit hyperactivity disorder (ADHD) in adults with LD

Key references

Amado H, Lustman P. Attention deficit disorder persisting in adulthood: a review. *Comprehensive Psychiatry* 1982; **23**: 300–314.

Aman MG, Marks RE, Turbot SH, Wilsher CP, Merry SN. Clinical effects of methylphenidate and thioridazine in intellectually sub-average children. *Journal of American Academic Child and Adolescent Psychiatry* 1991; **30**: 246–256.

Barkley RA. *Attention Deficit Disorder: A Handbook for Diagnosis and Treatment.* New York: Guilford Press, 1990, p. 47.

Barkley R, McMurray M, Edelbrock C, Robbins K. Side effects of methylphenidate in children with attention-deficit hyperactivity disorder: a systematic, placebo-controlled evaluation. *Pediatrics* 1990; **86**: 184–192.

Cantwell D. Genetics of hyperactivity. *Journal of Child Psychology and Psychiatry* 1975; **16**: 261–264.

Castellanos FX, Rapoport JL. Etiology of attention-deficit hyperactivity disorder. *Child and Adolescent Pediatric Clinics of North America* 1992; **1**: 373–384.

Fargason R, Ford C. Attention-deficit hyperactivity disorder in adults: diagnosis, treatment and prognosis. *Southern Medical Journal* 1994; **87**: 302–309.

Greenill L, Plizza S, Dulcan MK, Work Group on Quality Issues. Practice parameter for the use of stimulant medications in the treatment of children, adolescents and adults. *Journal of American Academic Child and Adolescent Psychiatry* 2002; **41**: 2.

Handen B, Johnson C, Lubitsky MJ. Efficacy of methylphenidate among children with autism and symptoms of attention deficit hyperactivity disorder. *Autism Developmental Disorders* 2000; **30**: 245–253.

Harris JC. The establishment of self-regulation and social understanding in children and adolescents with ADHD: family factors. In: Capute A, Accardo P, Shapiro B (eds). *Learning Disabilities Spectrum: ADD, ADHD and LD.* Baltimore, MD: York Press, 1994.

Lindsey M. Emotional, behavioural and psychiatric disorders in children. In: Russell O (ed). *Seminars in the Psychiatry of Learning Disabilities.* London: Royal College of Psychiatrists, 1997, p. 92.

MTA Co-operative Group. A 14 month randomised clinical trial of treatment strategies for attention-deficit/hyperactivity disorder. Multimodal treatment study of children with attention-deficit/hyperactivity disorder. *Archives of General Psychiatry* 1999; **56**: 1073–1086.

National Institute for Clinical Excellence. Guidance on the use of methylphenidate (Ritalin, Equasym) for attention deficit hyperactivity disorder (ADHD) in childhood. London: NICE, October 2000.

O'Malley A, Clark A. Diagnosis and management of ADHD in young adults. *Progress in Neurology and Psychiatry* 2003; **7**: 24–27.

Steingard R, Biedornan J, Spencer T, Wilens T, Gonzalez A. Comparison of clonidine response in the treatment of attention-deficit hyperactivity disorder with and without co-morbid tic disorders. *Journal of American Academic Child and Adolescent Psychiatry* 1993; **32**: 350–353.

Swanson J, McBurnett K, Wigel T et al. Effect of stimulant medication on children with attention deficit disorder: a 'review of reviews'. *Exceptional Children* 1993; **60**: 154–162.

chapter 9

Anxiety disorders

Definition

Anxiety disorders encompass a range of disorders in which the primary symptom is anxiety that is not secondary to a major psychiatric illness (such as depression) and *not* induced by substance abuse (ICD-10). Symptoms of anxiety may be broadly classified as follows:

- cognitive, that is, apprehension (worry about the future, feeling on edge and difficulty in concentrating)

- motor, as in restless fidgeting, tension headaches, trembling and inability to relax

- autonomic, as in dry mouth, dizziness, sweating, tachycardia, tachypnoea and epigastric discomfort.

Three major groups of anxiety disorders can be characterized.

Phobic anxiety disorder

Phobic anxiety is evoked by certain well-defined situations or objects that are not currently dangerous. As a result, these situations or objects are characteristically avoided or endured with dread. Phobic anxiety disorder includes agoraphobia, social phobia and specific phobias.

Obsessive compulsive disorder

The essential features of obsessive compulsive disorder (OCD) are recurrent obsessional thoughts and/or compulsive acts or rituals.

Other anxiety disorders

A number of other disorders are characterized by major symptoms of anxiety that are not restricted to any particular environmental situation. These include the following:

- **Panic disorder**: several severe attacks of autonomic anxiety occur within a period of 1 month with comparative freedom from symptoms between attacks.

- **Generalized anxiety disorder**: generalized and persistent anxiety is not restricted to any particular environmental circumstances, as in free-floating anxiety.

- **Mixed anxiety and depressive disorder**: both anxiety and depression are present, but neither is sufficiently severe to justify a diagnosis.

Prevalence

Within the general adult population, the prevalence of anxiety disorders varies between studies, although it is consistently higher in females. In the 1997 National Psychiatric Morbidity Survey, the point prevalence of any neurotic disorder was 19.5% in females and 17.3% in males; that of generalized anxiety disorder, 3.4% and 2.8%, respectively; that of phobias, 1.4% and 0.7%, respectively; and that of panic disorder, 0.9% and 0.8%, respectively.

A few studies suggest that there is a higher prevalence of anxiety disorders in adults with learning disability (LD) than in the general adult population. This may be due to decreased adaptive abilities, insufficient coping strategies, inadequate communication to express distress and/or low self-esteem. Anxiety may be difficult to diagnose because repetitive movements and behaviour are common in LD.

Key points specific to learning disability

Management of anxiety disorders

The management of anxiety disorders, including phobias and OCD, is predominantly based on psychotherapeutic approaches such as anxiety management training, cognitive behaviour therapy and other behavioural approaches (exposure and response prevention). Drug therapy should be considered only if behavioural approaches fail or if there are major co-morbid mental health problems.

Psychotherapeutic approaches for patients with LD are limited because of the restricted cognitive abilities of this patient group. Sometimes a combination of psychotherapeutic and pharmacological approaches is useful.

In general, drugs known to cause dependence, such as benzodiazepines, should be used only as a last resort. Their use should be limited to 4 weeks to avoid the development of physical dependence and tolerance.

Anxiety disorders in individuals with pervasive developmental disorders

Individuals with pervasive developmental disorders (PDD), such as autistic spectrum disorders (including Asperger's syndrome), are often anxious in social or communal settings due to their difficulty in reciprocating social and emotional cues. Anxiety may become even more pronounced if a fixed routine or pattern is disrupted. As a result of these individuals' underlying need for predictability, any changes in their life should be small enough to accustom them to the variation.

Phobias seen in individuals with PDD can be more bizarre and intense than those usually seen in the general adult population. This may be the result of unusual perception.

Stereotypy and repetitive behaviour are characteristic of autistic individuals. Although this behaviour may resemble the rituals exhibited by people with OCD, it is difficult to assess to what extent it is a source of comfort and pleasure. In addition, it may be difficult to elicit any obsessional thoughts producing the compulsions because of the individuals' limited ability to express themselves. Social anxiety is often more pronounced in those with Asperger's syndrome or with high-functioning autism.

Aggression is a frequent response to a perceived threat in many individuals with autism.

Anxiety and behaviour problems

Anxiety may be a cause of the sudden onset of behaviour problems in individuals with LD, particularly in those with moderate or severe LD. This may result from a lack of communication skills. People with LD may also be more sensitive to stress due to concomitant poor physical health, social isolation and/or environmental pressure. Studies using anxiolytics to control aggression provide indirect evidence for this. In severe behaviour problems, antipsychotics can be used as a last resort.

Anxiety and self-injurious behaviour

Anxiety may be a component of self-injurious behaviour associated with features of hyperarousal, autonomic hyperactivity and generalized behaviour disturbance. Anxiolytics and mood-stabilizing drugs have been used in this group of patients with benefit.

Obsessive compulsive disorder

The few studies that have been carried out for the symptomatic treatment of compulsive actions or rituals in people with LD show that clomipramine and selective serotonin re-uptake inhibitors (SSRIs) are effective.

Treatment

Obsessive compulsive disorder in adults with learning disability

Algorithm 9.1 should be used as a guide only for the treatment of adults with both LD and OCD.

Panic disorders in adults with learning disability

Algorithm 9.2 should be used as a guide only for the treatment of adults with both LD and panic disorders.

Generalized anxiety disorder in adults with learning disability

Algorithm 9.3 should be used as a guide only for the treatment of adults with both LD and generalized anxiety disorder.

Note 1: *propranolol*. Patients need to be monitored for bradycardia and hypotension. Contraindications to propranolol are asthma, heart failure, heart block and peripheral vascular disease.

Note 2: *benzodiazepines*. The use of benzodiazepines should be limited to a maximum of 4 weeks to avoid any physical dependence.

Note 3: *duration of treatment*. A good response to SSRIs and selective noradrenaline re-uptake inhibitors (SNRIs) is usually not sustained when the medication is withdrawn. A rebound phenomenon may be observed. If withdrawal is attempted, a gradual withdrawal is preferable to avoid discontinuation reactions, especially with short-acting SSRIs or SNRIs.

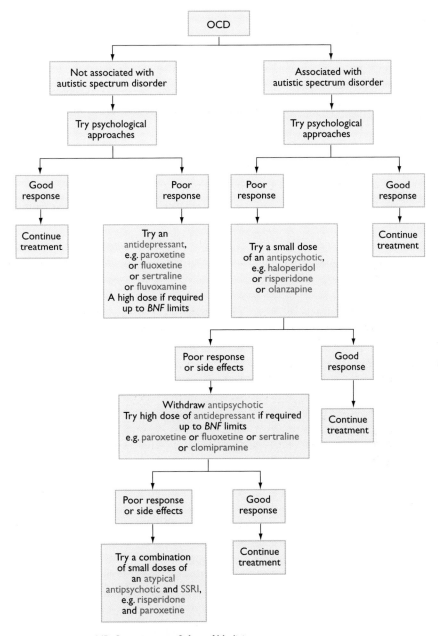

NB: Committee on Safety of Medicines
1. There is an increased risk of cerebrovascular adverse events in older patients with dementia treated with olanzapine or risperidone.
2. Please refer to caution regarding the use of SSRIs and SNRIs.

Algorithm 9.1 Treatment of obsessive compulsive disorder (OCD) in adults with LD

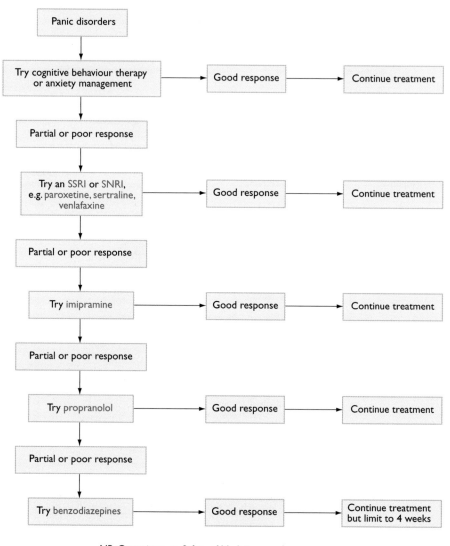

Panic disorders

Try cognitive behaviour therapy or anxiety management → Good response → Continue treatment

Partial or poor response

Try an SSRI or SNRI, e.g. paroxetine, sertraline, venlafaxine → Good response → Continue treatment

Partial or poor response

Try imipramine → Good response → Continue treatment

Partial or poor response

Try propranolol → Good response → Continue treatment

Partial or poor response

Try benzodiazepines → Good response → Continue treatment but limit to 4 weeks

NB: Committee on Safety of Medicines
1. There is an increased risk of cerebrovascular adverse events in older patients with dementia treated with olanzapine or risperidone.
2. Please refer to caution regarding the use of SSRIs and SNRIs.

Algorithm 9.2   Treatment of panic disorders in adults with LD

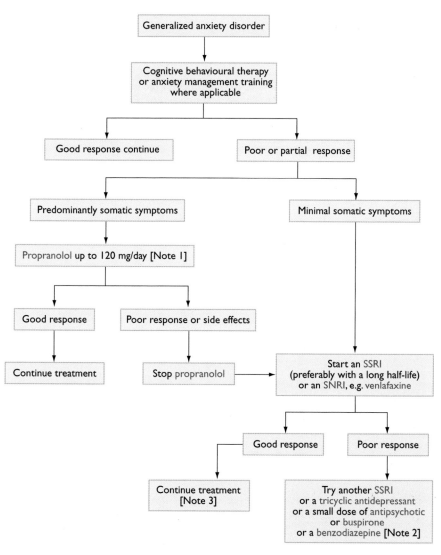

NB: Committee on Safety of Medicines
1. There is an increased risk of cerebrovascular adverse events in older
   patients with dementia treated with olanzapine or risperidone.
2. Please refer to caution regarding the use of SSRIs and SNRIs.

Algorithm 9.3 Treatment of generalized anxiety disorder in adults with LD

Key references

Jenkins R, Lewis G, Bebbington P et al. The National Psychiatric Morbidity Surveys of Great Britain—initial findings from the household survey. *Psychological Medicine* 1997; **27**: 775–789.

Kalachnick JE, Leventhal BL, James DH et al. Guidelines for the use of psychotropic medication. In: Reiss S, Aman MG (eds). *Psychotropic Medications and Developmental Disabilities. The International Consensus Handbook.* Columbus, OH: Ohio State University Press, 1998, pp. 45–72.

Werry JS. Anxiolytics and sedatives. In: Reiss S, Aman MG (eds). *Psychotropic Medications and Developmental Disabilities. The International Consensus Handbook.* Columbus, OH: Ohio State University Press, 1998, pp. 201–214.

Zarcone JR, Hellings JA, Crandall K et al. Effects of risperidone on aberrant behaviour of persons with developmental disabilities. I. A double-blind cross-over study using multiple measures. *American Journal of Mental Retardation* 2001; **106**: 525–538.

chapter 10

Affective disorders

Definition

Affective disorders are characterized by a change in mood or affect, usually to depression (with or without associated anxiety) or to elation (ICD-10). The mood change is generally accompanied by a change in the overall level of activity, and most other symptoms are secondary to this change. The disorders tend to be recurrent, and the onset of individual episodes is often related to a stressful event or situation.

Prevalence

Surveys within the general population have shown that the point prevalence of depression is around 2%; that of bipolar disorder, 1.5%; and that of all affective disorders, 2.8%. Surveys of patients in long-term institutional care have shown a higher prevalence of affective disorders (5.5%) than community surveys (2.3%). The lifetime prevalence of depression in the general population is 5–6%; that of bipolar disorder, 0.5–1.5%; and that of all affective disorders, 6–17%.

Studies of the point prevalence of depression in adults with learning disability (LD) show levels between 1.3% and 3.7%. Studies suggest that affective disorders, particularly depression, are often underdiagnosed and inadequately treated in people with LD. Older people with LD may be more prone to depression, with 8.9% of hospital residents and 6.7% of community residents affected.

Key points specific to learning disability

Presentation of depression

The diagnosis of affective disorder in people with LD is compounded by the difficulties arising from communication problems, the influence of poor physical and social circumstances and a general lack of suitable diagnostic criteria. Thus, the overall prevalence of depression in this population may be underestimated.

Depression of mood may be missed or misdiagnosed more frequently than hypomania or bipolar disorder in people with LD. The onset of depression tends to be more insidious and the changes less dramatic than in the general population. Symptoms are often attributed to the underlying LD or the onset of dementia.

Symptoms of depression include weepiness and social withdrawal. With increasing severity of LD, irritability may be much more marked and become the predominant expression of depression. Psychomotor agitation is also more common in those with more severe disabilities, whereas reduced energy and fatigue are more frequently seen in those with mild or moderate LD.

Biological symptoms of depression include changes in appetite and sleep pattern. Increased appetite with weight gain are as common as decreased appetite with weight loss. Insomnia is much more common than hypersomnia, particularly in those with more severe LD.

A wide variety of behavioural symptoms are associated with depressive illness. The most obvious include aggression, self-injurious behaviour, screaming, temper tantrums, stereotypes, incontinence and vomiting.

Aggression is a common symptom in depression, and has also been reported in both hypomania and rapid cycling bipolar disorder. The association with affective disorders is of great practical importance, as it can dominate the presentation. Carers and health-care professionals may be less likely to identify other features such as biological changes or changes in mood.

Hypochondriacal symptoms, such as headache, abdominal pain and vomiting, may be prominent in the presentation of depression.

Some individuals may present with a generalized deterioration in their social relationships and self-care skills. There is a high correlation between ratings for depression and social skills. There is therefore a risk that a diagnosis of dementia may be made and appropriate treatment withheld, particularly for older patients with Down syndrome.

The diagnosis of affective disorders in individuals with severe or profound LD is based mostly on reports of a change in behaviour (such as recent onset of emotional lability, irritability, weepiness or elevation of mood) from carers and/or a change in biological features (such as activity, sleep, appetite or sexual behaviour). Anxiety, a frequent co-morbid symptom, may be expressed in the form of avoidance behaviour or autonomic features in relation to a specific situation.

Uncommon symptoms of depression include erotomanic delusions and worsening of pica.

Depression and Down syndrome

Individuals with Down syndrome are more prone to depression than those with LD of other aetiologies (11% and 4%, respectively). Studies have also shown that those with Down syndrome and a past history of depression have significantly lower adaptive behaviour skills than others.

An early age of onset of depression in an individual with Down syndrome is a particularly poor prognostic indicator. Relapse of depression may be more common in those with a short duration of the index episode, the presence of biological symptoms of depression and a marked loss of interest in all pleasurable activities (anhedonia).

Mania and hypomania

Mania and hypomania in LD generally present with an increase in motor activity. Mood is less likely to be euphoric or infectious and more likely to be irritable and accompanied at times by aggression. While pressure of speech may be present, more complex verbal symptoms, such as flight of ideas or clang associations, are rare. Grandiose ideas and delusions are usually in a simple form, and hallucinations are rare.

Rapid cycling bipolar disorder (four or more episodes of affective illness in 1 year) is associated with severe behaviour problems in individuals with LD, particularly self-injurious behaviour.

Affective disorders and autism

In people with autistic spectrum disorders, diagnosing an affective disorder may be difficult against the background of autistic symptoms. Deterioration in cognition, language or behaviour is more common than a specific change in mood. Baseline values should be considered in evaluating any change in behaviour such as increased self-injury, echolalia or hand-clapping.

Affective disorders, epilepsy and learning disability

Brain damage associated with LD plays an important role in the aetiology of affective disorders in those with epilepsy. Antiepileptic drugs may lead to secondary depression.

Bereavement

For an individual with LD, bereavement may be a particularly threatening life event, especially if it results in rapid changes in personal circumstances. Intense reactions, such as self-injury, may be observed in as many as 10–15% of reactions to grief, and depressive symptoms are frequent.

Suicide

Although suicide is rarely reported in people with LD, suicidal behaviours, including threats of suicide and self-injurious behaviour with suicidal intent, have been described.

One study found that suicidal individuals tend to be young and to have borderline LD and chronic poor health or physical disability.

Drug treatment of depression

Efficacy and effectiveness of antidepressants

There are no systematic controlled drug trials of treatment of depression in people with LD. However, the existing literature of case reports and case series suggests that the efficacy and effectiveness of antidepressants in people with LD are very similar to those in the general population:

- The efficacies of selective serotonin re-uptake inhibitors (SSRIs) and of tricyclic antidepressants (TCAs) are similar.

- SSRIs are considered to be better tolerated than TCAs. TCAs may have unwanted side effects such as anticholinergic effects, postural hypotension and cardiac conduction disturbances.

- SSRIs are considered to be reasonably safe to use in conjunction with drugs such as lithium and carbamazepine.

Concerns about antidepressants

There are, however, the following concerns about using antidepressants in people with LD:

- Most antidepressants present a moderate risk of worsening seizures. The risk is *lower* with SSRIs and monoamine oxidase inhibitors (MAOIs) than with TCAs.

- Hypomania and increased maladaptive behaviours have been shown to emerge in up to a third of patients treated with SSRIs.

- There may be withdrawal problems on discontinuation, particularly with paroxetine.

Duration and ending of treatment

The duration of treatment for depression and the strategy for ending treatment should be the same as recommended for the general population:

- For the first episode of depression, maintenance treatment should be given for 6–9 months at the dose of antidepressant used to achieve full recovery.

- For recurrent depression, maintenance treatment should be given for 2–5 years at the dose of antidepressant used to achieve full recovery.

- Antidepressant treatment should be gradually withdrawn over a period of 4–6 weeks, using a tapering dose regimen to avoid discontinuation reactions.

Discontinuation reactions

Discontinuation reactions characteristically appear within a few days of stopping treatment and usually resolve within 2–4 weeks. Such reactions may be experienced after cessation of traditional TCAs as well as the newer SSRIs and serotonin and noradrenaline re-uptake inhibitors (SNRIs). They are more common after the abrupt cessation of antidepressants with a short half-life, such as paroxetine and fluvoxamine, and are rarely seen after cessation of those with a longer half-life, such as fluoxetine.

Discontinuation reactions usually consist of influenza-like symptoms (fever, nausea, vomiting, insomnia, headache and sweating) and, at times, anxiety and agitation. Discontinuation reactions to SSRIs may also include dizziness, vertigo and light-headedness, and occasionally sensory symptoms such as paraesthesia, numbness and the sensation of electric shocks.

Drug treatment of bipolar affective disorder

Lithium has been successfully used in the prophylaxis of bipolar disorder in LD. Lithium is generally well tolerated, although some side effects, such as tremors, weight gain and hypothyroidism, may be unacceptable. In addition, regular blood monitoring may prove to be difficult in some patients due to lack of understanding and cooperation. Other mood-stabilizing drugs, such as carbamazepine and sodium valproate, have also been shown to be effective.

Additional therapeutic drugs, such as antipsychotics and benzodiazepines, are frequently used in clinical practice to control behaviour symptoms associated with depression and hypomania. Although adjunctive treatment is necessary in many cases, there are risks of misdiagnosing the primary psychiatric disorder and of treatment being used for non-specific behaviour control. The latter may result in excessive use of tranquillizing medication, without optimal therapeutic benefit to the patient.

Cautionary notes regarding polypharmacy

Individuals with LD are more prone to drug interactions than the general population because more than one drug is usually prescribed. For a comprehensive description of common drug interactions in treating affective disorders, refer to the *British National Formulary*.

Treatment algorithms

Depression in adults with learning disability

Algorithm 10.1 should be used as a guide only for the treatment of adults with both LD and depression.

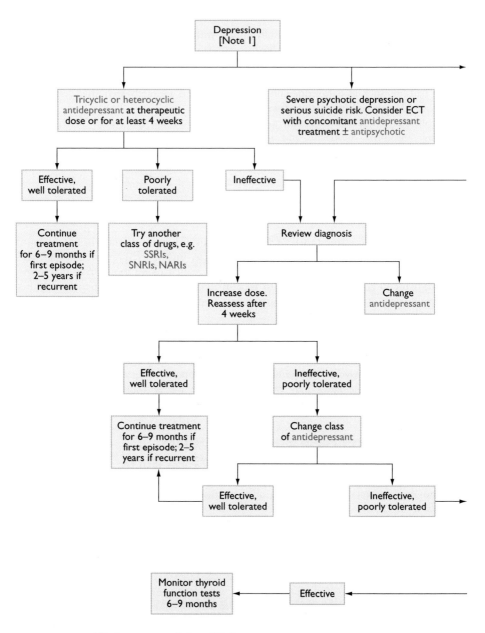

Depression
[Note 1]

Tricyclic or heterocyclic antidepressant at therapeutic dose or for at least 4 weeks

Severe psychotic depression or serious suicide risk. Consider ECT with concomitant antidepressant treatment ± antipsychotic

Effective, well tolerated

Poorly tolerated

Ineffective

Continue treatment for 6–9 months if first episode; 2–5 years if recurrent

Try another class of drugs, e.g. SSRIs, SNRIs, NARIs

Review diagnosis

Increase dose. Reassess after 4 weeks

Change antidepressant

Effective, well tolerated

Ineffective, poorly tolerated

Continue treatment for 6–9 months if first episode; 2–5 years if recurrent

Change class of antidepressant

Effective, well tolerated

Ineffective, poorly tolerated

Monitor thyroid function tests 6–9 months

Effective

NB: Committee on Safety of Medicines
1. There is an increased risk of cerebrovascular adverse events in older patients with dementia treated with olanzapine or risperidone.
2. Please refer to caution regarding the use of SSRIs and SNRIs.

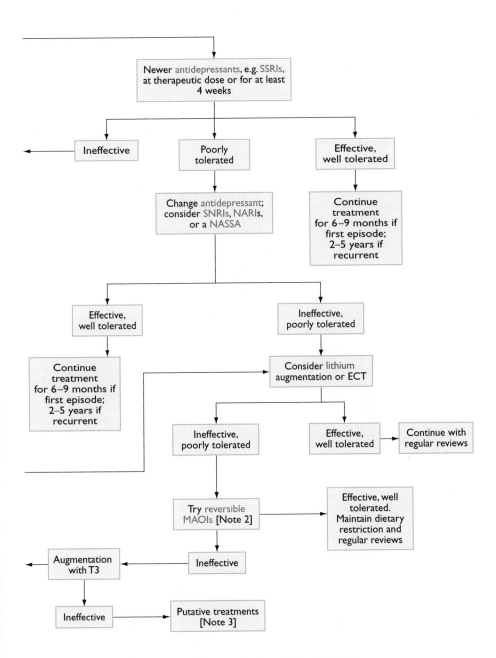

Algorithm 10.1 Treatment of depression in adults with LD

Note 1: *drug choice.* Drug treatment is indicated for all cases with moderate or severe depressive episodes. The choice of drug depends on the presence of any co-morbid psychiatric diagnoses (Table 10.1) and whether the patient falls into any special group (Table 10.2). The treatment of depression in adults with LD now mostly involves using the newer antidepressants because of their reduced incidence of side effects.

Note 2: *dietary restrictions.* There are fewer dietary restrictions with moclobemide than with other MAOIs, but the restrictions still apply.

Note 3: *putative treatments.* The following options may be considered if first-line treatments are unsuccessful (Table 10.3). A second opinion is advisable before considering putative treatments.

Table 10.1	Drug treatment of depression with other co-morbid psychiatric diagnoses
Co-morbidities	*Options for treatment*
Depression plus symptoms of anxiety	Paroxetine, sertraline, amitriptyline, fluoxetine, trazodone, citalopram, venlafaxine
Depression plus psychomotor retardation	Imipramine, fluoxetine, venlafaxine, reboxetine, lofepramine
Depression plus obsessive compulsive features	SSRIs, especially paroxetine TCAs, especially clomipramine
Depression plus psychotic symptoms	SSRIs with or without small doses of typical or atypical antipsychotics Electroconvulsive therapy (ECT) if indicated Venlafaxine
Depression plus bipolar affective disorder	SSRIs
Depression plus deliberate self-harm	SSRIs Venlafaxine

Table 10.2 Drug treatment of depression in special patient groups

Special patient groups	Drug choice in depression
Women of child-bearing age	SSRIs, especially fluoxetine, paroxetine
Pregnant women	SSRIs, especially fluoxetine Benefits to mother and risk to fetal weight depend on the trimester
Older persons	SSRIs, especially paroxetine, citalopram, sertraline Venlafaxine **Avoid** TCAs and reboxetine
People with Down syndrome	SSRIs
People with epilepsy	SSRIs Consider moclobemide, other MAOIs, reboxetine, tryptophan Adjust dose of antiepileptic drug if necessary **Avoid** TCAs
People with cardiovascular problems	SSRIs **Avoid** TCAs, especially dosulepin (dothiepin)

Table 10.3 Putative treatments for depression

Putative treatment options	Cautions
High doses of venlafaxine up to 300 mg/day	Has the potential to lower blood pressure Monitor blood pressure
Add lithium in adequate doses to achieve a serum concentration of 0.4–0.6 mmol/l	Monitor plasma levels and toxic side effects
Add tryptophan 6–9 g/day in divided doses to the antidepressant	Risk of serotonin syndrome Special registration requirements
Add lamotrigine of up to 200 mg/day in divided doses to the antidepressant	Titrate the dose gradually
High dose of TCA, e.g. imipramine 300 mg/day	Electrocardiogram monitoring of cardiac side effects is essential
Combine a TCA with a MAOI, e.g. phenelzine	Extreme caution: serious drug interaction
Combine ECT with antidepressant medication	Short-term memory disturbances

Mania and hypomania

Algorithm 10.2 should be used as a guide only for the treatment of adults with both LD and mania or hypomania. This incorporates guidance from the National Institute for Clinical Excellence on the use of olanzapine and sodium valproate in the treatment of acute mania associated with bipolar disorder.

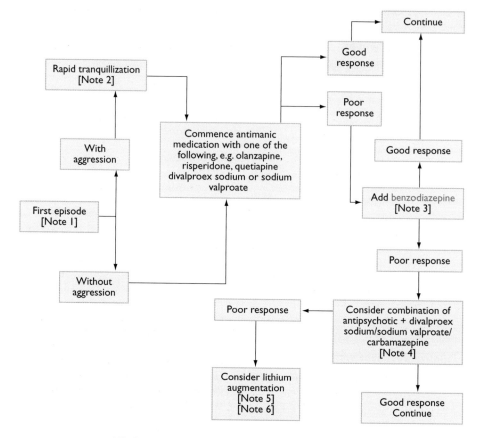

NB: Committee on Safety of Medicines
1. There is an increased risk of cerebrovascular adverse events in older patients with dementia treated with olanzapine or risperidone.
2. Please refer to caution regarding the use of SSRIs and SNRIs.

Algorithm 10.2 Treatment of first episode of mania/hypomania in adults with LD

Note 1: *first episode*. In the acute treatment of the first episode of mania and hypomania, antipsychotic medication alone or in combination with a benzodiazepine has been found to be effective. Treatment should be given for between 6 months and 1 year.

Note 2: *rapid tranquillization*. Rapid tranquillization may be required during the acute excitement phase. Haloperidol 5–10 mg IV or IM is first given with lorazepam 1–2 mg IM stat. This may be followed after an interval of at least 30 min by the same combination of drugs as initially or by a benzodiazepine alone. In a 24-h period, the maximum dose of haloperidol that should be given is 18 mg, and that for lorazepam is 4 mg. If further sedation is required, it is preferable to prescribe a benzodiazepine at the same time as beginning an oral antipsychotic and mood stabilizer (except in the first episode). Zuclopenthixol acetate may be a useful adjuvant to consider.

Note 3: *duration of treatment.* The use of benzodiazepines should be restricted to 4 weeks to avoid the risk of physical dependency.

Note 4: *other mood-stabilizing drugs.* The two common mood-stabilizing drugs used instead of lithium are as follows:

- carbamazepine: starting with 100–200 mg/day and gradually increasing the dose according to the response

- sodium valproate: starting with 200 mg twice a day and gradually increasing the dose according to the response.

Note 5: *contraindications to lithium.* Lithium is teratogenic and carries a 1 in 1000 risk of causing Ebstein's anomaly. Therefore, whenever possible, lithium should be avoided during pregnancy, especially in the first trimester. However, the decision to prescribe lithium should be made after weighing the risk of relapse against the risk of causing a fetal abnormality. One option may be to reduce the dose of lithium until the least effective dose is reached. During the later stages of pregnancy, the dose may need to be increased due to the increased maternal renal clearance and fluid volume. Serum lithium levels should be monitored at least once a month throughout pregnancy and more frequently in the third trimester. Adequate water and salt intake must be maintained throughout pregnancy. Thyroid function must be monitored. Patients should be advised to report symptoms of toxicity immediately. Lithium is contraindicated in Addison's disease, in renal or cardiac disease, and during lactation. In people with epilepsy, therapeutic doses of lithium may induce electroencephalogram (EEG) changes. It may also lower the seizure threshold, resulting in generalized tonic-clonic and myoclonic seizures. Co-administration with carbamazepine or phenytoin may predispose to neurotoxicity, which is associated with seizures. It has been found that pre-existing EEG abnormalities, concomitant antipsychotic medication, cerebral disorder and genetic susceptibility predispose to **lithium toxicity**.

Note 6: *monitoring lithium levels.* The serum lithium concentration for prophylaxis is 0.4–0.8 mmol/l. The dose of lithium may be adjusted to achieve this. The optimum dose varies among individuals. During lithium prophylaxis, the serum concentration should be monitored every 2–3 months. The baseline investigations (note 3) should be repeated every 6 months. Lithium prophylaxis should ideally last 3–4 years, but therapy should be continued only if the benefits persist.

Note 7: *prophylaxis.* Before beginning treatment with a mood-stabilizing drug, **baseline investigations** should be done as follows: full blood count; urea and electrolyte levels; liver function tests; thyroid function tests; and electrocardiogram (ECG).

Lithium treatment should not be started unless serum levels can be monitored. The serum lithium concentration should be measured 1 week after starting treatment and weekly thereafter until the concentration is 0.6–1.0 mmol/l. Lithium may be started at the same time as an oral antipsychotic, and the antipsychotic may be stopped at a later date. Alternatively, mood may be initially stabilized by an antipsychotic, and lithium may be started later, followed by a gradual cessation of the antipsychotic.

Treatment of mania/hypomania bipolar affective disorder in adults with LD

Algorithm 10.3 should be used as a guide only for the treatment of adults with both LD and bipolar affective disorder.

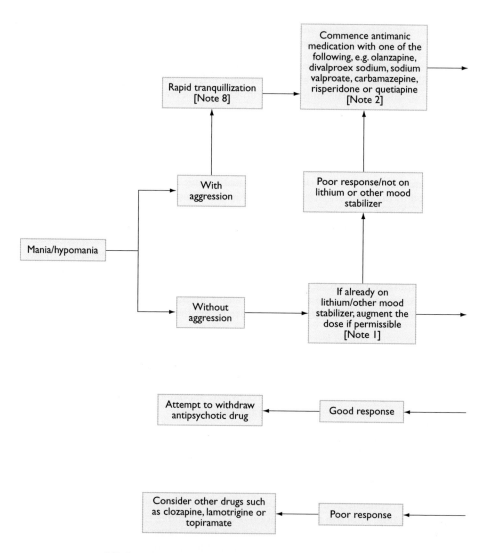

NB: Committee on Safety of Medicines
1. There is an increased risk of cerebrovascular adverse events in older patients with dementia treated with olanzapine or risperidone.
2. Please refer to caution regarding the use of SSRIs and SNRIs.

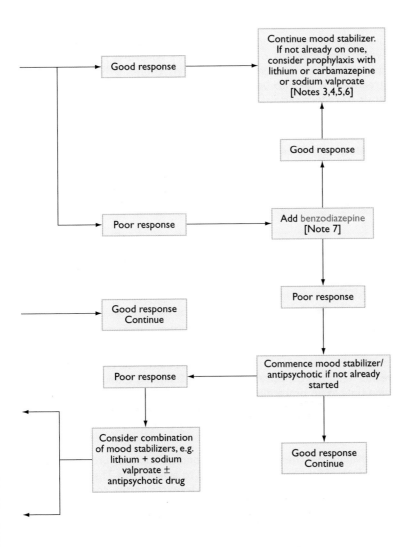

Good response

Continue mood stabilizer. If not already on one, consider prophylaxis with lithium or carbamazepine or sodium valproate [Notes 3,4,5,6]

Good response

Poor response

Add benzodiazepine [Note 7]

Good response
Continue

Poor response

Poor response

Consider combination of mood stabilizers, e.g. lithium + sodium valproate ± antipsychotic drug

Commence mood stabilizer/ antipsychotic if not already started

Good response
Continue

Algorithm 10.3 Treatment of mania/hypomania associated with bipolar affective disorder in adults with LD

Note 1: *acute treatment.* During an acute attack of mania or hypomania, lithium treatment may take 10 days or more to exert its antimanic effect; therefore, concomitant treatment with a benzodiazepine or an antipsychotic is usually required. Alternatively, a low dose of haloperidol or a benzodiazeipine is often used as the treatment of choice. The dose of antipsychotic medication should be kept low if co-prescribed with lithium, because high doses of typical antipsychotics, such as haloperidol, fluphenazine or flupentixol, have been known to cause irreversible toxic encephalopathy when used concomitantly with lithium.

Note 2: *atypical antipsychotics.* Atypical antipsychotics may be used to control the initial manic or hypomanic symptoms, or when psychotic symptoms persist, or when the patient develops side effects with conventional antipsychotics. When the duration of antipsychotic treatment is likely to be prolonged, it is preferable to change to an atypical antipsychotic to reduce the risk of serious side effects such as tardive dyskinesia.

Note 3: *prophylaxis.* Before beginning treatment with a mood-stabilizing drug, **baseline investigations** should be done, as set out in the box:

Baseline investigations

- full blood count
- urea and electrolyte levels
- liver function tests
- thyroid function tests
- electrocardiogram (ECG).

Lithium treatment should not be started unless serum levels can be monitored. The serum lithium concentration should be measured 1 week after starting treatment and weekly thereafter until the concentration is 0.6–1.0 mmol/l. Lithium may be started at the same time as an oral antipsychotic, and the antipsychotic may be stopped at a later date. Alternatively, mood may be initially stabilized by an antipsychotic, and lithium may be started later, followed by a gradual cessation of the antipsychotic.

Note 4: *monitoring lithium levels.* The serum lithium concentration for prophylaxis is 0.4–0.8 mmol/l. The dose of lithium may be adjusted to achieve this. The optimum dose varies among individuals. During lithium prophylaxis, the serum concentration should be monitored every 2–3 months. The baseline investigations (note 3) should be repeated every 6 months. Lithium prophylaxis should ideally last 3–4 years, but therapy should be continued only if the benefits persist.

Note 5: *other mood-stabilizing drugs.* The two common mood-stabilizing drugs used instead of lithium are as follows:

- carbamazepine: starting with 100–200 mg/day and gradually increasing the dose according to the response

- sodium valproate: starting with 200 mg twice a day and gradually increasing the dose according to the response.

Note 6: *contraindications to lithium.* Lithium is teratogenic and carries a 1 in 1000 risk of causing Ebstein's anomaly. Therefore, whenever possible, lithium should be avoided during pregnancy, especially in the first trimester. However, the decision to prescribe lithium should be made after weighing the risk of relapse against the risk of causing foetal abnormality. One option may be to reduce the dose of lithium until the least-effective dose is reached. During the later stages of pregnancy, the dose may need to be increased due to the increased maternal renal clearance and fluid volume. Serum lithium levels should be monitored at least once a month throughout pregnancy and more frequently in the third trimester. Adequate water and salt intake must be maintained throughout pregnancy. Thyroid function must be monitored. Patients should be advised to report symptoms of toxicity immediately. Lithium is contraindicated in Addison's disease, in renal or cardiac disease, and during lactation. In people with epilepsy, therapeutic doses of lithium may induce EEG changes. It may also lower the seizure threshold, resulting in generalized tonic-clonic and myoclonic seizures. Co-administration with carbamazepine or phenytoin may predispose to neurotoxicity, which is associated with seizures. It has been found that pre-existing EEG abnormalities, concomitant antipsychotic medication, cerebral disorder and genetic susceptibility predispose to **lithium toxicity.**

Note 7: *duration of treatment.* The use of benzodiazepines should be restricted to 4 weeks to avoid the risk of physical dependency.

Note 8: *rapid tranquillization.* Rapid tranquillization may be required during the acute excitement phase. Haloperidol 5–10 mg IV or IM is first given with lorazepam 1–2 mg IM stat. This may be followed after an interval of at least 30 min by the same combination of drugs as initially or by a benzodiazepine alone. In a 24-h period, the maximum dose of haloperidol that should be given is 18 mg, and that for lorazepam is 4 mg. If further sedation is required, it is preferable to prescribe a benzodiazepine at the same time as beginning an oral antipsychotic and mood stabilizer (except in the first episode). Zuclopenthixol acetate may be a useful adjuvant to consider.

Rapid-cycling mood disorder in adults with learning disability

Algorithm 10.4 should be used as a guide only for treatment of adults with both LD and rapid-cycling mood disorder. Rapid-cycling mood disorder refers to four of more episodes of mood disorder in a year.

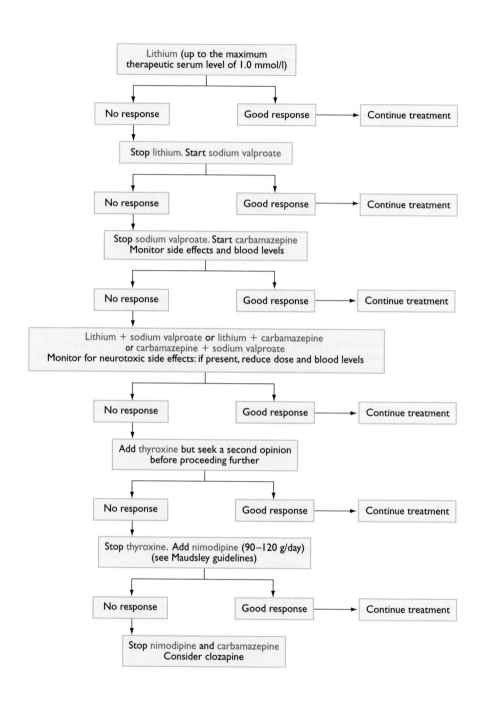

Algorithm 10.4   Treatment of rapid-cycling mood disorder in adults with LD

Schizoaffective disorder in adults with learning disability

Algorithm 10.5 should be used as a guide only for the treatment of adults with both LD and schizoaffective disorder.

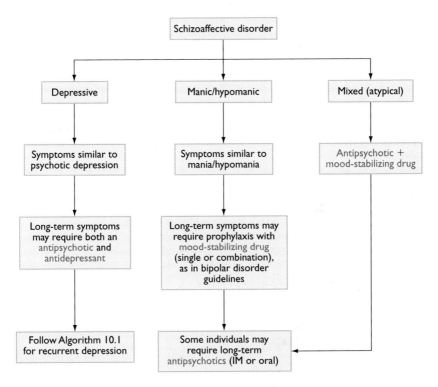

NB: The presence of prominent affective and schizophrenic symptoms may need treatment for both schizophrenia and affective disorder (see Algorithms 11.1 and 10.1). Single episodes require short-term treatment, but recurrent episodes will require long-term treatment, with a need to review the diagnosis on a regular basis.

NB: Committee on Safety of Medicines
1. There is an increased risk of cerebrovascular adverse events in older patients with dementia treated with olanzapine or risperidone.
2. Please refer to caution regarding the use of SSRIs and SNRIs.

Algorithm 10.5 Treatment of schizoaffective disorder in adults with LD

Key references

Anderson IM, Edwards JG. Guidelines for choice of selective serotonin re-uptake inhibitor in depressive illness. *Advances in Psychiatric Treatment* 2001; **7**: 170–180.

Barbui C, Hotopf M, Freemantle N et al. SSRIs versus tricyclic antidepressants: comparison of drug adherence. *Cochrane Database of Systematic Reviews*. Oxford: 2002.

Bauer MS, Whybrow PC. Rapid cycling bipolar affective disorder. II. Treatment of refractory rapid cycling with high dose levothyroxine: a preliminary study. *Archives of General Psychiatry* 1990; **47**: 435–440.

Bhaumik S, Branford D, Naik BI, Biswas AB. Retrospective audit of selective serotonin re-uptake inhibitors (fluoxetine and paroxetine) of the treatment of depressive episodes in adults with learning disability. *British Journal of Developmental Disabilities* 2000; **46**: 131–139.

Biswas AB, Bhaumik S, Branford D. Treatment emergent behavioural side effects with selective serotonin re-uptake inhibitors in adults with learning disabilities. *Human Psychopharmacology* 2001; **16**: 133–137.

Bowden CL, Brugger AM, Swann AC et al. Efficacy of valproate versus lithium and placebo in the treatment of mania. *JAMA* 1994; **27**: 18–24.

Calabrese JR, Bowden CL, Sachs GS, Ascher JA, Monaghan E, Rudd GD. A double blind placebo controlled study of lamotrigine monotherapy in outpatients with bipolar I depression. Lamictal 602 Study Group. *Journal of Clinical Psychiatry* 1999; **60**: 79–88.

Calabrese JR, Delnechi GA. Spectrum of efficacy of valproate in 55 patients with rapid cycling bipolar disorder. *American Journal of Psychiatry* 1990; **147**: 431–434.

Dubovsky SL. Calcium channel antagonists as novel agents for manic depressive disorder. In: Schatzburg AF, Nerneroff CB (eds). *Textbook of Psychopharmacology*. Washington, DC: American Psychiatric Press, 1995, pp. 455–472.

Hotopf M, Lewis G, Normand C. Are SSRIs a cost-effective alternative to tricyclics? *British Journal of Psychiatry* 1996; **168**: 404–409.

Howland R. Fluoxetine treatment of depression in mentally retarded adults. *Journal of Nervous and Mental Disease* 1992; **180**: 202–205.

Langee HR, Conlon M. Predictors of response to antidepressant medications. *American Journal of Mental Retardation* 1992; **97**: 65–70.

Maj M, Pirozzi R, Magliano L, Baroli L. Long-term outcome of lithium prophylaxis in bipolar disorder: a 5-year prospective study of 402 patients at a lithium clinic. *American Journal of Psychiatry* 1998; **155**: 30–35.

Masi G, Marchesci M, Pfanner P. Paroxetine in depressed adolescents with intellectual disability—an open label study. *Journal of Intellectual Disability Research* 1997; **41**: 268–272.

Sovner R, Pay RJ, Dosen A et al. Antidepressants. In: Reiss S, Aman MG (eds). *Psychotropic Medications and Developmental Disabilities. The International Consensus Handbook*. Columbus, OH: Ohio State University Press, 1998, pp. 179–200.

Tohen M, Sanger TM, McElroy SL et al and the Olanzapine HGEH Group. Olanzapine versus placebo in the treatment of acute mania. *American Journal of Psychiatry* 1999; **156**: 702–709.

chapter 11

Schizophrenia

Definition

Schizophrenia is described as an enduring mental illness characterized by the presence of delusions, hallucinations and distortion of thinking and perception—with or without negative symptoms—of at least 6 months' duration that tends to cause significant social and/or occupational dysfunction and is *not* attributable to substance abuse or an organic condition (DSM-IV).

Prevalence

The prevalence of schizophrenia in the general population is 2.5–5.3 per 1000. The prevalence of schizophrenia in the learning disability (LD) population depends on the nature of the study sample. The prevalence is 3.2–3.4% in hospital samples and 1.3–3.0% in community samples. The prevalence of schizophrenia is highest in those with a mild degree of LD, decreasing with a decrease in level of intelligence (IQ) (Table 11.1).

Table 11.1 Prevalence of schizophrenia in adults with LD

Severity of LD	IQ	Prevalence
Mild	50–69	3.3%
Moderate	35–49	2.6%
Severe	20–34	1.2%
Profound	<20	0%

Key points specific to learning disability

Atypical presentations

Schizophrenia may manifest itself atypically in people with LD. If positive symptoms predominate, the individual is likely to suffer from simple hallucinations in the form of noises. Similarly, delusional beliefs tend to have simple themes that are somewhat fantastic. Individuals with a limited ability to communicate may present with hallucinatory behaviour or with extremely disturbed behaviour that is out of character for them. Those with predominantly negative symptoms may present with a regression of their skills and symptoms such as lack of motivation. These may be difficult to identify, particularly in those who are recipients of passive care.

Limited language skills

It is difficult to diagnose schizophrenia reliably in people with limited language skills. The diagnosis may be easier in those with a mild degree of LD if sufficient allowance is made for their reduced vocabulary. However, as the criteria used in both operational schedules ICD-10 and DSM-IV are based on language, a diagnosis of schizophrenia is unlikely to be made with confidence in individuals with an IQ of less than 50.

Behaviour impairment

Many individuals with LD may have a concomitant behaviour disorder, which may confound a diagnosis of schizophrenia. This is particularly the case when major impairment of social interaction is a valid criterion.

Affective disorders and negative symptoms

Affective disorders are not uncommonly seen in people with LD and schizophrenia. Depression, side effects of antipsychotic drugs and the primary cause of LD may prevent a confident diagnosis of negative symptoms.

Schizophrenia and epilepsy

About 20–30% of individuals with LD and schizophrenia also have concomitant epilepsy. In these individuals, it is important to remember the possible confounding factors caused by the use of psychotropic and antiepileptic drugs. It may be difficult to make a clinical diagnosis of schizophrenia confidently, especially in the presence of postictal symptoms. Similarly, there is considerable overlap of affective symptoms and the negative symptoms of schizophrenia. This may be complicated by issues related to the side effects of antipsychotic drugs and the primary cause of the LD. Schizophrenic symptoms seen ictally and postictally, especially those in temporal lobe epilepsy, need to be differentiated from those associated with interictal schizophrenia. Phenomena such as kindling, forced normalization and lowering of the seizure threshold may be observed.

Monitoring progress and response to treatment

Rating scales such as the Clinical Interview Schedule, the Psychopathology Inventory for Mentally Retarded Adults (PIMRA) and the Diagnostic Assessment for the Severely Handicapped (DASH) rely on interview and carer information. This may not be robust when following up the response to treatment in those with LD. Difficulties in monitoring the progression of illness may be complicated by clinician bias and unreliable assessments of the dose and duration of medication.

Treatment

The National Institute for Clinical Excellence (NICE) has produced guidelines for the core interventions in the treatment of schizophrenia in the general population. The following guidance is based on these recommendations with adaptations for use in the LD population. Clinicians should evaluate the tolerance and efficacy of current treatments against new antipsychotics as they become available.

Neurotoxicity

People with LD are likely to develop side effects with antipsychotics due to their underlying brain damage. Neurological side effects are most common, particularly extrapyramidal side effects such as Parkinsonism, dystonia, akathisia (restlessness), tardive dyskinesia and, rarely, neuroleptic malignant syndrome. However, some abnormal neurological movements may present premorbidly in some individuals due to their underlying brain damage. Therefore, it is important to monitor neurological side effects on a regular basis as routine practice, using scales such as the Abnormal Involuntary Movement Scale (AIMS). People with LD are also likely to experience other side effects, such as QTc prolongation, hepatic impairment and blood dyscrasia, due to their multisystem impairment. The monitoring of side effects relies on carer involvement. Monitoring by periodic investigation may prove difficult in some patients due to their lack of understanding and cooperation.

Cognition

There is good evidence in adults with normal intelligence that antipsychotics may cause sedation, psychomotor impairment and decreased ability to concentrate. These effects may be compounded in adults with LD because of the underlying organic condition.

Drug interactions

Co-morbidity, such as a physical illness or epilepsy, results in multiple drug regimes for the majority of people with LD. This increases their risk of drug interactions. Some of the important drug interactions are given in Table 11.2. The *British National Formulary* (*BNF*) should be consulted for more detailed information.

Table 11.2 Common drug interactions in people with LD being treated for schizophrenia

Drug combination	Common interactions
Antipsychotics plus lithium	Increasing lithium levels has a **direct neurotoxic effect**, including neuroleptic malignant syndrome, particularly with clozapine, haloperidol and phenothiazine
Antipsychotics plus antiepileptics	The **threshold for convulsions** is lowered Carbamazepine **accelerates the metabolism** (that is, reduces the plasma concentration) of clozapine, haloperidol, olanzapine and risperidone Phenytoin **accelerates the metabolism** (that is, reduces the plasma concentration) of clozapine and quetiapine The risk of **neutropenia** is increased if olanzapine is given with sodium valproate
Antipsychotics plus antidepressants	Increased risk of **arrhythmia** with tricyclic antidepressants Selective serotonin re-uptake inhibitors and venlafaxine increase the **plasma concentration** of clozapine Fluoxetine increases the **plasma concentration** of haloperidol Nefazodone increases the **plasma concentration** of haloperidol
Antipsychotics plus antiarrhythmic drugs	Increased risk of **ventricular arrhythmia** with antiarrhythmic drugs that prolong the QT interval such as amiodarone, disopyramide, procainamide and quinidine
Antipsychotics plus angiotensin-converting enzyme inhibitors or calcium channel blockers	Risk of **postural hypotension**
Antipsychotics plus cimetidine	Cimetidine increases the **plasma concentration** of many antipsychotic drugs, including clozapine
Chlorpromazine plus propranolol	Chlorpromazine may increase the **plasma concentration** of both itself and propranolol

Algorithm 11.1 should be used as a guide only for the treatment of adults with LD and co-existing schizophrenia or other psychotic disorders. The use of depot antipsychotics is omitted from the figure. Depot preparations may be considered when compliance is an issue, and for individuals suspected of being fast metabolizers. However, there is a risk of tardive dyskinesia after long-term use, with the probable exception of atypical depot preparations such as Risperdal Consta.

Cautionary note

Ideally, only one antipsychotic should be prescribed at any given time, and it is generally unacceptable for more than two antipsychotics to be prescribed concurrently. However, if two antipsychotics are required, the rationale for such a prescription should be clearly documented in the patient's notes. The patient should be monitored regularly for side effects and for the effects of drug interactions. If the prescription of more than two classes of psychotropic medication is considered necessary, a second opinion is advisable.

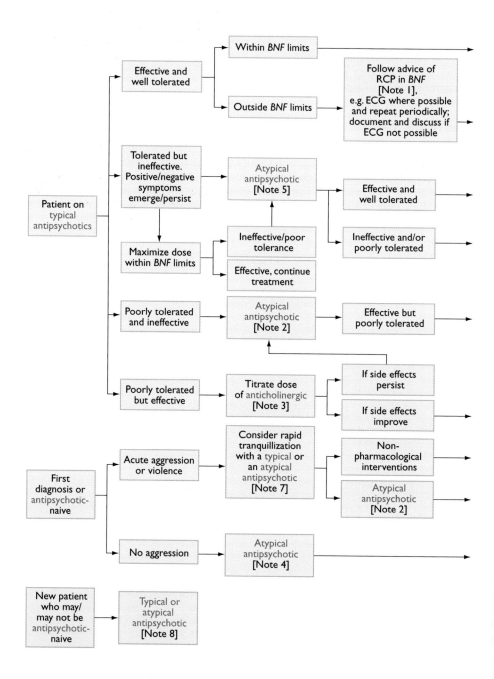

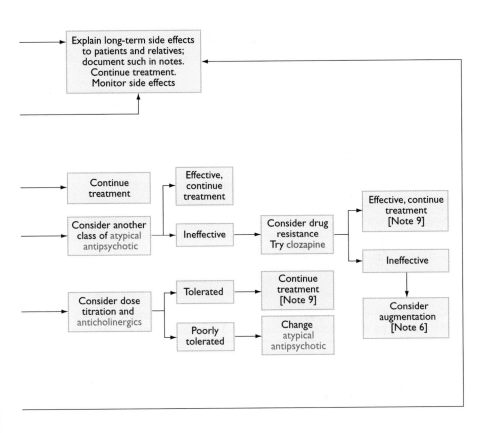

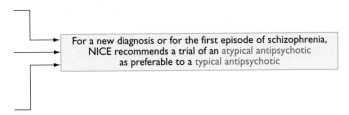

NB: Committee on Safety of Medicines
1. There is an increased risk of cerebrovascular adverse events in older
   patients with dementia treated with olanzapine or risperidone.
2. Please refer to caution regarding the use of SSRIs and SNRIs.

Algorithm 11.1 Drug treatment of schizophrenia and other psychotic orders in adults with LD

Note 1: *high doses*. Advice about using antipsychotics above the doses in the *BNF* has been provided by the Royal College of Psychiatrists (RCP) (box).

Royal College of Psychiatrists' advice on doses above *BNF* upper limit

1 Consider alternative approaches, including adjuvant therapy and newer or atypical antipsychotics such as clozapine.

2 Bear in mind risk factors, including obesity—particular caution is indicated in older patients, especially those over 70.

3 Consider the potential for drug interactions—consult the *BNF*.

4 Carry out an electrocardiogram (ECG) to exclude any untoward abnormalities such as a prolonged QT interval. Repeat ECGs periodically and reduce the dose if a prolonged QT interval or another adverse abnormality develops.

5 Increase the dose slowly, and not more often than once weekly.

6 Carry out regular pulse, blood pressure and temperature checks, and ensure that the patient maintains adequate fluid intake.

7 Consider high-dose therapy to be for a limited period. Review regularly. Abandon if no improvement occurs after 3 months (return to standard dose).

If an ECG cannot be carried out due to lack of patient cooperation, this should be documented in the patient's notes. The maximum tolerated dose may be given for 3–4 weeks before changing the drug.

Note 2: *atypical antipsychotics* (Table 11.3).

Table 11.3	Common effects of atypical antipsychotics compared with typical antipsychotics	
	Typical antipsychotics	**Atypical antipsychotics**
Advantages	Efficacy is the same as that of atypical antipsychotics Low cost	Fewer acute extrapyramidal side effects; clozapine and olanzapine in particular cause fewer cases of tardive dyskinesia Most have a lower potential for reducing the seizure threshold than typical antipsychotics (see exceptions below) Clozapine, olanzapine and quetiapine do not elevate the prolactin concentration as much as other antipsychotics

Table 11.3 *Continued*

	Typical antipsychotics	Atypical antipsychotics
Disadvantages	More acute extrapyramidal side effects especially akathisia; higher long-term risk of tardive dyskinesia Epileptogenecity is well recognized Long-term use of thioridazine in high doses may cause retinitis pigmentosa Neuroleptic malignant syndrome has been reported	Risperidone at high doses (>4 mg/day) is as likely as typical antipsychotics to cause acute extrapyramidal side effects Clozapine and zotepine are epileptogenic Olanzapine has an increased risk of causing hyperglycaemia and hyperlipidaemia; need to monitor blood glucose and lipid profile Weight gain is common, notably with olanzapine Neuroleptic malignant syndrome has been reported

Changing from a typical antipsychotic to an atypical antipsychotic has been found to reduce the subjective symptoms of akathisia and hypokinesia. Where weight gain is a problem, amisulpride, quetiapine or zotepine should be considered. Clinicians should consult the Committee on Safety of Medicines for further information about neuroleptic malignant syndrome.

Note 3: *anticholinergics*. Anticholinergic drugs should not be prescribed for more than 4 weeks. If the patient requires anticholinergics on a regular basis or for longer than 4 weeks, it may indicate drug intolerance and warrant either a change in dose or choice of drug. If extrapyramidal side effects of an antipsychotic are severe, it is preferable to change the medication to one better tolerated than to treat with anticholinergics. Anticholinergics should be withdrawn gradually.

Note 4: *efficacy of atypical antipsychotics*. Atypical antipsychotics are considered to be as effective as typical antipsychotics in the treatment of positive symptoms. Clozapine has been found to be effective in the treatment of refractory psychosis and negative symptoms. Risperidone, quetiapine, amisulpride and olanzapine have also been found to be useful in the treatment of negative symptoms.

Note 5: *switching antipsychotics*. There is no consensus on how to switch antipsychotics. It should be noted that antipsychotics may produce gastric side effects, particularly those with inherent muscarinic activity. Many antipsychotics have long elimination half-lives, particularly in depot formulation, and switches may take many weeks or months. The *BNF* provides guidance of equivalent doses when making a switch.

Note 6: *augmentation strategies*. Augmentation strategies include lithium for schizoaffective symptoms, carbamazepine for aggression and sodium valproate for mood disturbance. Clozapine should *not* be used concurrently with carbamazepine due to drug interactions. If augmentation strategies fail, consider unproven therapies such as the following:

- clozapine plus amisulpride
- clozapine plus small doses of risperidone or amisulpride or haloperidol
- a course of electroconvulsive therapy.

The patient's consent should be obtained wherever possible. Therapy should be documented in the patient's notes and continued for a fixed period of 3–4 weeks with frequent evaluation.

Note 7: *rapid tranquillization*. Atypical antipsychotics may be used to control the initial manic or hypomanic symptoms or when psychotic symptoms persist, or when the patient develops side effects with conventional antipsychotics. When the duration of antipsychotic treatment is likely to be prolonged, it is preferable to change to an atypical antipsychotic to reduce the risk of serious side effects such as tardive dyskinesia.

Note 8: *special patient groups*. Compared with typical antipsychotics, atypical antipsychotics put patients at a lower risk of short-term side effects. However, long-term experience of atypical antipsychotics is limited. Even at low doses of antipsychotics, older people are more likely to develop extrapyramidal symptoms, particularly with typical antipsychotics. The preferred drugs for each subject group are shown in Table 11.4.

Table 11.4 Drug treatment of schizophrenia in special patient groups

Special patient groups	Drug choice in schizophrenia
Women of child-bearing age	Low dose of an antipsychotic, provided there is no hindrance to conception by raising prolactin levels If medication is essential, chlorpromazine or trifluoperazine may be prescribed There is no conclusive evidence to support the safety of atypical antipsychotics Manufacturers advise *against* amisulpride, and recommend olanzapine, risperidone or quetiapine *only if* the potential benefits outweigh the risks
Pregnant women	*Avoid* all antipsychotics in the first trimester *Avoid* risperidone and amisulpride if hyperprolactinaemia is symptomatic
Lactating women	*Avoid* all antipsychotics unless absolutely necessary Chlorpromazine appears to be safest but causes drowsiness in the infant
Young and middle-aged men	Olanzapine, risperidone, quetiapine or amisulpride Monitor weight gain and hyperprolactinaemia, particularly with risperidone and amisulpride *Avoid* risperidone and amisulpride if hyperprolactinaemia is symptomatic Use quetiapine for those who have acute dystonia with other antipsychotics

Table 11.4 *Continued*	
Special patient groups	**Drug choice in schizophrenia**
Older men and women	Olanzapine, risperidone or amisulpride in low doses Begin slowly and increase slowly while monitoring side effects frequently NB: Committee on Safety in Medicine warning: there is an increased risk of cerebrovascular adverse events in older patients with schizophrenia when treated with olanzapine or risperidone
Obese men and women	*Avoid* olanzapine and chlorpromazine; preference for amisulpride or quetiapine

Note 9: *duration of treatment.* The duration of treatment depends on patient response. After the first episode, treatment should be for at least a 2-year symptom-free period, ideally with one antipsychotic medication.

Key references

Bethlem and Maudsley NHS Trust. *Maudsley 2003 Prescribing Guidelines.* London: Martin Dunitz, 2003.

Corbett J. Psychiatric morbidity and mental retardation. In: Smith P, James FE (eds). *Psychiatric Illness and Mental Handicap.* Ashford: Headley Brothers, 1979, pp. 11–25.

Duggan L, Brylewski J. *Antipsychotic Medication for Those with Both Schizophrenia and Learning Disability (Cochrane Review).* Oxford: Cochrane Library Issue 3, update software, 1998.

Duggan L, Brylewski J. Effectiveness of antipsychotic medication in people with intellectual disability and schizophrenia: a systematic review. *Journal of Intellectual Disability Research* 1999; **43**: 94–104.

Heaton-Ward WA. Psychosis in mental handicap. *British Journal of Psychiatry* 1977; **130**: 524–533.

Jablensky A. Epidemiology of schizophrenia: a European perspective. *Schizophrenia Bulletin* 1986; **12**: 52–73.

Kalachnik JE, Leventhal BL, James DH et al. Guidelines for the use of psychotropic medication. In: Reiss S, Aman MG (eds). *Psychotropic Medications and Developmental Disabilities. The International Consensus Handbook.* Columbus, OH: Ohio State University Press, 1998, pp. 45–47.

Lund J. The prevalence of psychiatric morbidity in mentally retarded adults. *Acta Psychiatrica Scandinavica* 1985; **72**: 563–570.

Menolascino FJ, Ruedrich SL, Wilson TE (1985). Diagnosis and pharmacotherapy of schizophrenia in the retarded. *Psychopharmacology Bulletin* 1985; **21**: 316–322.

National Institute of Clinical Excellence. *Clinical Guideline 1 Schizophrenia. Core Interventions in the Treatment and Management of Schizophrenia in Primary and Secondary Care.* London: NICE, 2002.

Reid AH. Psychosis in adult mental defectives. *British Journal of Psychiatry* 1972; **120**: 205–218.

Sijatortic M, Ramirez LF, Kenny JT, Meltzer HY. The use of clozapine in borderline intellectual functioning and mentally retarded schizophrenic patients. *Comprehensive Psychiatry* 1994; **35**: 29–33.

Wright EC. The presentation of mental illness in mentally retarded adults. *British Journal of Psychiatry* 1982; **141**: 496–502.

chapter 12

Personality disorders

Definition

Personality disorders are defined in ICD-10 as 'deeply ingrained and enduring behaviour patterns, manifesting themselves as inflexible responses to a broad range of personal and social situations. They represent either extreme or significant deviations from the way the average individual in a given culture perceives, thinks, feels and particularly relates to others. Such behavioural patterns tend to be stable and to encompass multiple domains of behaviour and psychological functioning. They are sometimes associated with various degrees of subjective distress and problems in social functioning and performance.'

Personality disorders fall broadly into three major clusters, each with a number of types (Table 12.1).

Table 12.1 Classification of personality disorders in ICD-10 and DSM-IV

Clusters	ICD-10	DSM-IV
Eccentric/odd	Paranoid Schizoid	Paranoid Schizoid Schizotypal
Flamboyant/dramatic	Dissocial Emotionally unstable: impulsive type borderline type Histrionic	Antisocial Borderline Histrionic Narcissistic
Anxious/fearful	Anankastic (obsessive-compulsive) Anxious (avoidant) Dependent	Obsessive-compulsive Avoidant Dependent
Other	Other	Passive-aggressive

The diagnosis of personality disorders in people with learning disability (LD) is contentious. Paranoid, schizoid, anxious and explosive personality types were identified in people with LD in a large population-based survey, but the largest category of personality disorders comprises impulsive or immature behaviour patterns. A systematic study looked at people with mild and moderate LD resident in hospital. It showed that personality disorders presented predominantly with mood symptoms in females and with explosiveness or aggressiveness in males. A classification of personality types based on more developmental concepts is generally considered more appropriate for people with more severe LD.

Prevalence

Population-based studies show that the prevalence of behaviour/personality disorders in people with LD is 22–25%. Around 7–10% of adults with LD who make up the caseload of specialist community mental health teams have a personality disorder. In forensic settings, the prevalence of personality disorder is 60–90%.

Key points specific to learning disability

Diagnosis

Though contentious, the diagnosis of personality disorders in people with LD is clinically relevant because it affects many aspects of management. It may be a determining factor in an individual's acceptability in a non-hospital environment. In routine clinical practice, the diagnosis of personality disorder is limited to people with mild or moderate LD. The diagnosis of personality disorders becomes more difficult in those with severe or profound LD. Considerable doubt also remains about the extent to which a diagnosis of challenging behaviour in this group overlaps with that of personality disorders.

Symptoms

A preliminary study exploring predominant symptom domains in a community sample of adults with LD and personality disorders described behaviour dyscontrol/aggression in 93%, mood dysregulation in 77%, deliberate acts of self-harm in 52%, psychotic symptoms in 47% and anxiety in 33%. Antipsychotics were used in 86%, antidepressants in 45%, mood-stabilizing drugs in 21% and anxiolytics in 10%.

Sexual behaviour

Problems of sexuality and sexual behaviour occur in adults with LD and can be very persistent and resistant to treatment. Such problems predominantly arise among adults with mild LD but also occasionally occur in those with more severe disabilities. Sexual exploitation and an inability to find appropriate sexual partners may occasionally lead to prostitution and paedophilia. In most people with LD, problems of sexual behaviour are most appropriately seen as developmental phenomena and as socially inappropriate rather than as driven by deviant or aberrant sexuality. Common examples of socially inappropriate sexual behaviour include excessive physical affection and masturbation in public. These problems are best treated through education, counselling or a behavioural approach.

Treatment

Although no drug has been licensed specifically for the treatment of personality disorders, psychotropic medication is widely used in clinical practice to relieve the disruption and distress caused to themselves and others by patients with personality disorders. However, research suggests that better outcomes may be obtained by combining pharmacological and psychological treatments.

The literature on drug treatments for personality disorders in adults with LD is limited and mostly comprises case series or small retrospective surveys.

Drug treatment of personality disorders may be based on clinical diagnosis but is more usefully done by a target symptom domains approach. This is based on the Temperament-Character-Intelligence model of personality and is reflected in the guidelines from the American Psychiatric Association for the treatment of borderline personality disorder.

Treatment based on clinical diagnosis

Eccentric personality disorders

There is very little evidence about the effectiveness of antipsychotics or other psychotropic drugs in treating patients with paranoid or schizoid personality disorder.

Flamboyant personality disorders

Low doses of haloperidol or thiothixene are effective in reducing typical borderline behaviour and associated symptoms, including depression. However, improvements do not seem to last beyond 16 weeks. There may be problems with adverse effects and poor compliance even with small doses.

Selective serotonin re-uptake inhibitors (SSRIs) may be useful in reducing impulsiveness and deliberate self-harm, and fluoxetine in reducing anger. Studies comparing tricyclic antidepressants, particularly amitriptyline, give conflicting results, and it has been suggested that there are different kinds of borderline personality disorder that respond differently to therapy. Monoamine oxidase inhibitors (MAOIs), such as phenelzine and tranylcypromine, may also be effective in borderline personality disorder.

Low doses of antipsychotics, including depot preparations, have been recommended for many years for the treatment of antisocial personality disorder. Lithium has been shown to reduce anger and impulsiveness in some of these patients.

Anxious/fearful personality disorders

There is difficulty in interpreting data from studies of patients with anxious personality disorders because the beneficial effects of a drug may result from its effects on mood rather than personality. There is also a problem of diagnostic overlap, particularly between avoidant personality disorder and social phobia. However, antidepressants in general seem to have some value in treatment and are widely used. Benzodiazepines have also been used. Gradual withdrawal is recommended if benzodiazepines have been given regularly for more than a few weeks.

Treatment based on symptom domains

The predominant symptom domains have been adapted for use in personality disorders in people with LD (Table 12.2). The different domains are not mutually exclusive, and in treating a patient it may be necessary to target more than one domain.

Table 12.2 Symptom domains used for treating personality disorders in people with LD

Domains	Main symptoms to be targeted
I Behaviour dyscontrol/ aggression/impulsivity	● Affective aggression: impulsive, hot-tempered behaviour associated with mood changes and often normal electroencephalogram (EEG) ● Predatory aggression: hostility, cruelty ● Organic-like aggression ● Ictal aggression: often associated with epilepsy and abnormal EEG
II Mood dysregulation	● Mood swings or mood instability ● Dysthymia-like symptoms or emotional detachment
III Anxiety symptoms	● Predominant cognitive anxiety ● Predominant somatic anxiety
IV Psychotic symptoms	● Chronic low-level symptoms ● Acute symptoms
V Acts of deliberate self-harm	● Self-harm

Algorithm 12.1 should be used as a guide only for the treatment of adults with both LD and a personality disorder. It follows the targeting of a predominant symptom domain approach. Treatment of aggression is considered in more detail in Chapter 6, and treatment of anxiety in Chapter 9.

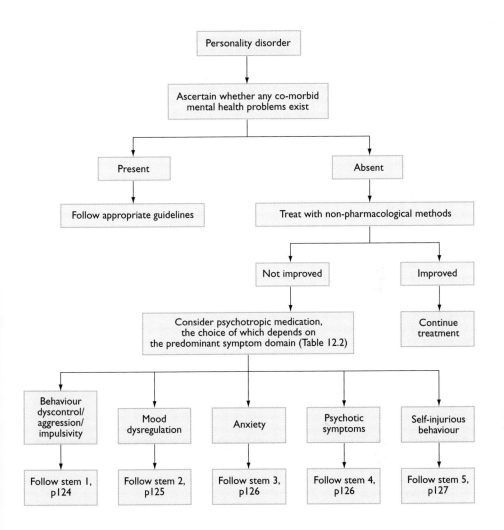

Algorithm 12.1   Treatment of personality disorders in adults with LD

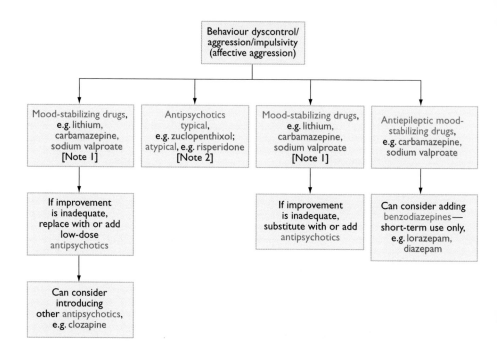

NB: Committee on Safety of Medicines
1. There is an increased risk of cerebrovascular adverse events in older patients with dementia treated with olanzapine or risperidone.
2. Please refer to caution regarding the use of SSRIs and SNRIs.

Algorithm 12.1 Treatment of personality disorders in adults with LD *continued*: stem 1

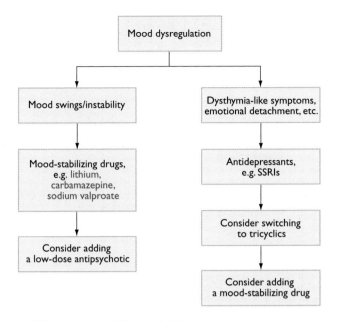

NB: Committee on Safety of Medicines
1. There is an increased risk of cerebrovascular adverse events in older patients with dementia treated with olanzapine or risperidone.
2. Please refer to caution regarding the use of SSRIs and SNRIs.

Algorithm 12.1 Treatment of personality disorders in adults with LD *continued*: stem 2

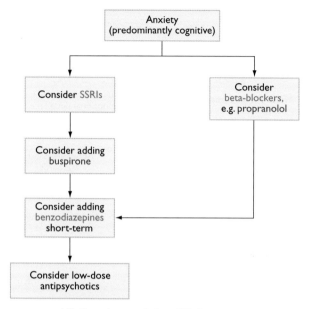

NB: Committee on Safety of Medicines
1. There is an increased risk of cerebrovascular adverse events in older patients with dementia treated with olanzapine or risperidone.
2. Please refer to caution regarding the use of SSRIs and SNRIs.

Algorithm 12.1 Treatment of personality disorders in adults with LD *continued*: stem 3

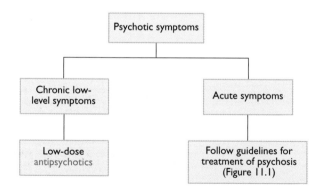

Algorithm 12.1 Treatment of personality disorders in adults with LD *continued*: stem 4

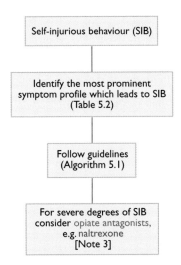

Self-injurious behaviour (SIB)

Identify the most prominent
symptom profile which leads to SIB
(Table 5.2)

Follow guidelines
(Algorithm 5.1)

For severe degrees of SIB
consider opiate antagonists,
e.g. naltrexone
[Note 3]

Algorithm 12.1 Treatment of personality disorders in adults with LD *continued*: stem 5

Note 1: *lithium*. There may be practical difficulties in obtaining blood tests for adequate monitoring, although some studies support the use of lithium in personality disorders, particularly in dealing with aggression. Drugs such as carbamazepine or sodium valproate may need to be used instead.

Note 2: *antipsychotics*. There are inadequate data to recommend any specific antipsychotic. Although there is some randomized, controlled-trial evidence for the usefulness of zuclopenthixol tablets, many clinicians prefer atypical antipsychotics because they have fewer side effects.

Note 3: *opiate antagonists*. The use of opiate antagonists, such as naltrexone, has been reviewed in the guidelines from the American Psychiatric Association on the management of deliberate self-harm in patients with borderline personality disorder.

Key references

Alexander R, Cooray S. Diagnosis of personality disorders in learning disability. *British Journal of Psychiatry* 2003; **182**: 28–31.

Esbensen AJ, Benson BA. Integrating behavioural, psychological and pharmacological treatment—a case study of an individual with borderline personality disorder and mental retardation. *Mental Health Aspects of Developmental Disabilities* 2003; **6**: 107–113.

Mavromatis M. The diagnosis and treatment of borderline personality disorder in persons with developmental disability—3 case reports. *Mental Health Aspects of Developmental Disabilities* 2000; **3**: 89–97.

Sadock BJ, Sadock VA. *Kaplan and Sadock's Synopsis of Psychiatry*, 9th edition. Philadelphia: Lippincott, Williams and Wilkins, 2003, pp. 819–821.

Schulz SC, Camlin KL. Risperidone for borderline personality disorder: a double-blind study. *Proceedings of the 39th Annual Meeting of the American College of Neuropsychopharmacology.* Nashville, TN: ACNP, 1999.

Soloff BH. Is there any drug treatment of choice for a borderline patient? *Acta Psychiatrica Scandinavica* 1994; **89**: 50–55.

Tyrer P. Drug treatment of personality disorder. *Psychiatric Bulletin* 1998; **22**: 242–244.

chapter 13

Ethnic variations in psychopharmacology

Total drug effect

The total effect of any drug on an individual depends on the pharmacological properties of that drug, the dose and the method of administration, the biological and psychological characteristics of the individual, and social and cultural factors. Chapter 1 describes how physical stature, physiology and brain damage in people with learning disability may affect the pharmacokinetics and efficacy of psychotropic drugs. This chapter focuses on how biological and cultural factors in different ethnic groups may lead to variations in the response to psychotropic medication.

Pharmacogenetics

There are variations between ethnic groups in the genes that code for the enzymes that metabolize drugs. These variations probably evolved in response to exposure to potentially harmful natural substances in the environment. Genetic variability within a population, including the capacity to handle a wide variety of toxic substances, is vital for its survival. Diversity across populations allows adaptation to different habitats.

Such genetic polymorphisms include genes that code for the following:

● synaptic receptors such as those for the monoamines, including noradrenaline, dopamine and serotonin

● transporting compounds that remove neurotransmitters from synapses

● enzymes involved in the metabolism and excretion of drugs.

Drug metabolism and cytochrome P450 enzymes

Most drugs are metabolized by liver enzymes, although some are destroyed by enzymes in the plasma or other tissues. Liver metabolism has two phases: phase I involves oxidation, reduction or hydrolysis; phase II involves conjugation. Differences in drug bioavailability due to liver metabolism are nearly always due to individual and genetic differences in the enzymes involved in phase I. Most commonly, this is the availability and range of cytochrome P450 enzymes, including the relatively scarce NADPH-cytochrome P450 reductase and the abundant cytochrome P450 terminal oxidase.

Several isoenzymes of P450 have been identified in man (Table 13.1). The CYP 3A family is present in the largest amounts and responsible for the metabolism of the greatest number of drugs. CYP 2D6, which accounts for less than 2% of the total P450 in the liver, is involved in the metabolism of many drugs.

Some isoenzymes have mutant alleles that function less efficiently than normal; around 50 have been identified for CYP 2D6. These may be categorized into the following four broad types of metabolizers:

- poor or ultraslow—no functioning gene; the individual is unable to produce the enzyme

- intermediate or slow—homozygotic or heterozygotic for one of the less efficient alleles

- extensive—two normally functioning alleles

- ultrarapid—three or more normally functioning alleles caused by multiplication.

The distribution of these phenotypes varies in different ethnic populations.

Table 13.1 Cytochrome P450 enzymes in relation to drug metabolism in the liver

Cytochrome P450 (CYP) enzymes	Metabolizes	Induced by	Inhibited by	Ethnic variations
CYP 1A2	Antipyrine Imipramine Clomipramine Clozapine Olanzapine Propranolol Theophylline	Smoking tobacco High-protein diet Cruciferous vegetables Aromatic hydrocarbons Cooking St John's wort	Fluvoxamine High-carbohydrate diet	
CYP 2C9	Warfarin Tolbutamide Losartan	St John's wort		Within total UK population $\leq 30\%$ slow metabolizers
CYP 2C19	Citalopram Diazepam Imipramine Omeprazole Phenytoin			Absent in: 3–5% Caucasians 23–30% Asians Slow metabolizers: 3–6% Caucasians 8–23% Asians
CYP 2D6	A large proportion of drugs including, codeine, β-blockers and tricyclic antidepressants, particularly: nortriptyline		Fluoxetine Paroxetine Haloperidol	Japanese and Chinese have the ultraslow phenotype and are particularly sensitive to drugs whose metabolism is mediated by this enzyme Absent in 7% Caucasians Absent in 1–2% non-Caucasians 7% in USA have genetic defect → the ultraslow metabolizer phenotype Within total UK population: $\leq 10\%$ slow metabolizers $\leq 10\%$ ultraslow metabolizers

131

Table 13.1 _Continued_

Cytochrome P450 (CYP) enzymes	Metabolizes	Induced by	Inhibited by	Ethnic variations
	clozapine olanzapine risperidone sertraline			Hyperactive in 30% of East Africans
CYP 3A3 **CYP 3A4**	The largest number of drugs, including: most calcium channel blockers most benzodiazepines most HMG-CoA-reductase inhibitors most nonsedating antihistamines ciclosporin cisapride clozapine quetiapine sertindole ziprasidone	Carbamazepine Rifabutin Rifampicin Troleandomycin St John's wort	Cimetidine Clarithromycin Erythromycin Troleandomycin Fluconazole Itraconazole Ketoconazole Most HIV protease inhibitors Fluvoxamine Nefazodone Norfluoxetine Grapefruit juice	

Non-genetic biological factors

The expression of drug-metabolizing enzymes may be affected by nutrients, plant products, drugs and other external chemical substances, and by endogenous hormones such as steroids. The cytochrome P450 enzymes CYP 1A2 and CYP 3A4 are most commonly induced or inhibited by these substances.

People from different ethnic backgrounds tend to have different lifestyles. These expose them to different substances that may affect the metabolism of any medication they take. For example, studies have shown that Asian Indians and Africans living in their native country and eating the local diet were significantly slower in metabolizing antipyrine, clomipramine and theophylline (involving CYP 1A2) than European Caucasians. After migrating to Europe and adopting the high-protein Western diet, the migrants' metabolic profiles for these drugs resembled those of the native Europeans.

CYP 3A4 acting at the steroid and xenobiotic receptors (SXR) provides a mechanism for rapidly detoxifying potentially harmful chemicals. Activating this SXR-CYP 3A4 system significantly enhances the removal of large foreign molecules. Inhibition of CYP 3A4 may increase the blood levels of certain drugs (Tables 13.1 and 13.2), potentially causing severe side effects.

Table 13.2 Some common effects of diet and tobacco on drug-metabolizing enzymes

Enzyme system	Diet or substance	Pharmacological effect
CYP 1A2	High-protein diet	Induces CYP 1A2
	Cruciferous vegetables such as cabbage, Brussels sprouts Aromatic hydrocarbons such as charboiled beef	Reduces blood concentration of: antipyrine, clomipramine, imipramine, clozapine, propranolol, theophylline
	High-carbohydrate diet	Inhibits CYP 1A2 Raises blood concentration of: antipyrine, clomipramine, theophylline
	Smoking tobacco	Reduces blood concentration of: most antipsychotic drugs by 50% most antidepressants by 50%
SXR-CYP 3A4	Grapefruit juice	Raises blood concentrations of: alprazolam, nefazodone, antiviral agents

However, there is no simple relationship between the plasma concentration of a drug and its therapeutic effects. The intersubject bioavailability of many psychotropic drugs is more than 50%, and with drugs such as paroxetine, no dose-response level has been demonstrated.

Significant herb–drug interactions may occur with St John's wort (*Hypericum perforatum*), a popular herbal remedy for mild depression. Preparations of St John's wort can induce drug-metabolizing enzymes, and a number of important interactions have been reported with many conventional drugs (Table 13.3). The amount of active ingredient varies between preparations, and switching from one to another may change the degree of enzyme induction. When an individual stops taking St John's wort, plasma concentrations of the conventional drug may increase, leading to toxicity.

Table 13.3 Drug interactions and precautions advised with St John's wort (SJW)

Drug	Effect	Precaution
Antiepileptics	Reduced plasma concentration carbamazepine, phenobarbital, phenytoin	Avoid concomitant use
Antiviral drugs	Reduced plasma concentration, e.g. indinavir by 57%	Avoid concomitant use
Calcium channel blockers	Reduced plasma concentration, e.g. nifedipine by 50%	Avoid concomitant use
Ciclosporin	Reduced plasma concentration of ciclosporin	Avoid concomitant use
Digoxin	Reduced plasma concentration of digoxin	Avoid concomitant use
Oral contraceptives	Reduced contraceptive effect	Avoid concomitant use
Selective serotonin re-uptake inhibitors	Increased serotonergic effects	Avoid concomitant use
Telithromycin	Reduced plasma concentration of telithromycin	Avoid while taking and for 2 weeks after stopping SJW
Theophylline	Reduced plasma concentration of theophylline	Avoid concomitant use
Warfarin	Reduced anticoagulant effect	Avoid concomitant use

Socio-cultural factors

Socio-cultural factors have a significant and often overlooked impact on the process of prescribing drugs. Pharmacotherapy can be understood in terms of a process of social transaction, which may be influenced by many factors, including the following:

- attributes of the drug itself: its taste, size, shape, colour, method of administration, packaging and name

- attributes of the patient: personality, socio-cultural background, experience, education and mental state
- attributes of the doctor: personality, status, authority, professional ideology, training and experience
- attributes of the setting: type of place, prescribing guidelines, wider policies and financial constraints
- influences of the pharmaceutical industry.

The complexity of influences on the total drug effect often results in wide individual and cultural variations in response to the same drug.

Both the patient and doctor are likely to be influenced by their own cultural beliefs about the world and how they perceive, interpret and understand reality, especially the occurrence of misfortunes such as illness and the role of prominent people within the society as healers. In some societies, the world-view is rationalistic; in others, it is more mystical. But each culture has its own healing rituals, such as the doctor–patient consultation in Western medicine.

The drug itself is a powerful symbol; and specific features, such as its colour and shape, can influence expectation in different ways in different cultures. In one study, white capsules were seen as analgesics by Caucasians and as stimulants by African-Americans. Different cultures have their preferred routes of administration.

The patient is also likely to be influenced by family members and friends, by relevant past experience and by the nature of the doctor–patient relationship. Rapport, mutual confidence and understanding between patient and doctor facilitate a patient's decision to accept and comply with treatment.

Socio-cultural factors also influence drug compliance. A South African study of 406 patients found that only 33% of black patients complied with treatment compared with 50% of Asian-Indian patients and 75% of white patients. The understanding of the treatment protocols was poor in the relatives of black and Asian-Indian patients compared with that of the relatives of white patients. Clear communication and understanding of socio-cultural factors are vital for effective treatment.

The placebo effect can be understood as the total drug effect without the presence of the drug. The *beliefs* of the patient (and doctor) in the *efficacy* of the placebo may have both psychological and physiological effects. The placebo effect may be an essential component of all forms of healing and therapy across cultures. However, placebos are administered in a specific social and cultural setting that validates both the placebo and the person administering it. Thus, placebos that work in one cultural group may not have any effect in another. The contribution of the placebo effect to the overall effectiveness of a pharmacologically active drug may also vary between different ethnic groups with different cultures.

The effects of globalization include rapid dissemination of information, cultural diffusion and homogenization of health beliefs and practices. However, indigenous medical concepts and practices remain between the different ethnic and cultural groups within a society, and need due consideration.

Key references

Aklillu E, Herrlin K, Gustafsson LL, Bertilsson L, Ingleman-Sunberg M. Evidence for environmental influence on CYP2D6-catalysed debrisoquine hydroxylation as demonstrated by phenotyping and genotyping of Ethiopians living in Ethiopia or in Sweden. *Pharmacogenetics* 2002; **12**(5): 375–383.

Ereshefsky L. Pharmacologic and pharmacokinetic considerations in choosing an antipsychotic. *Journal of Clinical Psychiatry* 1999; **60** (Suppl): 20–30.

Guengerich FP, Shimada T, Yun C-H et al. Interactions of ingested food, beverage and tobacco components involving human cytochrome P4501A2, 2A6, 2E1 and 3A4 enzymes. *Environmental Health Perspectives* 1994; **102** (suppl 9): 49–53.

Hasegawa M, Gutierrez-Esteinou R, Way L, Melzer HY. Relationship between clinical efficacy and clozapine concentrations in plasma in schizophrenia: effect of smoking. *Journal of Psychopharmacology* 1993; **6**: 383–390.

Perry PJ, Miller DD, Arndt SV, Smith DA, Holman TL. Haloperidol dosing requirements: the contribution of smoking and nonlinear pharmacokinetics. *Journal of Clinical Psychopharmacology* 1993; **13**: 46–51.

Shimada T, Yamazaki H, Mimura M, Inui Y, Guengerich FP. Individual variations in human liver cytochrome P-450 enzymes involved in oxidation of drugs, carcinogens and toxic chemicals: studies with liver microsomes of 30 Japanese and 30 Caucasians. *Journal of Pharmacology and Experimental Therapeutics* 1994; **270**: 414–423.

Summary of syndromes mentioned in the guidelines

Syndrome	Incidence	Aetiology/ genetics	Severity LD	Main features
Aicardi syndrome	200 cases by 1997	X-linked dominant	Severe	Agenesis of corpus callosum, severe visual defects (choroidoretinal lacunae), infantile spasms with associated abnormal EEG (hypsarrhythmia), skeletal abnormalities especially of ribs and spine. Usually presents in infants. Progressive course with psychomotor slowing, kyphoscoliosis, visual failure and typically death by early adulthood.
Cornelia de Lange syndrome	1:40 000– 1:100 000	Uncertain: most sporadic cases	Moderate/ severe	Typical facies (upturned nose, anteverted nostrils, arched eyebrows, long eyelashes, crescent-shaped mouth, long philtrum, high palate, micrognathia); limb abnormalities, failure to thrive due to gastro-oesophageal reflux (may lead to aspiration pneumonia and death). Autistic behaviours, especially stereotypies. Limited speech: a few words. Small stature, self-injury, undescended testicles, eye abnormalities.
Down syndrome	1:600	Trisomy 21	Mild/ moderate	Typical facies (upward-outward slanting eyes, epicanthus, wide nasal bridge), short stature, hyperflexia, gastrointestinal and congenital heart abnormalities. Hypertonia in childhood becomes less marked with age. Failure to thrive in infancy replaced by predisposition to obesity after age 3. Hearing impairments common. Language/speech deficits independent of LD level. Alzheimer's disease changes after age 35.
Fragile X syndrome	1:1000 – 1:2600 males	Distal arm Xq27.3 associated with FMR-1 gene	Mild/ moderate	Absence of FMR protein delays neuronal development. Females show less severe LD, milder phenotypic features and slower deterioration than males. Typical facies (macrocephaly, long face, large, prominent ears). Connective tissue disorder may contribute to heart defects and infections. Autistim-like behaviours, socially anxious, disturbed by a variety of stressors and environmental changes.

Syndrome	Incidence	Aetiology/genetics	Severity LD	Main features
Gilles de la Tourette syndrome	Incidence?	Obscure; involves hereditary factors and basal ganglia	Severity?	Multiple motor and vocal tics occurring many times a day (usually in bouts) most days or intermittently over 1 year or more. Onset before 18 years, usually 5–8 years. Tics usually affect facial muscles first and later spread to affect muscles of neck, trunk, arms and, rarely, legs. May also be coprolalia, echolalia, attention problems, fidgetiness, disinhibition, obsessive-compulsive behaviours and autistic features.
Lennox–Gestaut syndrome	Incidence? males	Uncertain	Moderate/severe	Combination of generalized seizures (atypical absences, tonic seizures, atonic attacks, myoclonic seizures); interictal EEG shows diffuse slow (2–3 Hz) spike and wave changes with bursts of fast activity (10 Hz) during sleep; slow mental development, often progressive LD.
Lesch–Nyhan syndrome	1:380 000	X-linked recessive	Mild/moderate	Inborn error of purine metabolism results in raised uric acid; untreated, this results in severe aggression, self-injury and gout. The risk of profound LD and self-injury relates to the degree of enzyme deficiency. Also severe motor disability, dystonia, growth retardation, visual impairments, feeding problems, involuntary movements, hypotonia, seizures. Early death from renal or respiratory failure or infection.
Phenylketonuria (PKU)	1:5000– 1:14 000	Autosomal recessive	Moderate/severe	Absence of phenylalanine hydroxylase causes inability to metabolize phenylalanine. A phenylalanine-free diet from first few weeks prevents LD. Inadequate dietary control may result in agitation, restlessness, intention tremor; tics. Neuropsychiatric symptoms arise if untreated.
Prader–Willi syndrome	1:10 000	Abnormal paternal 15q11–13 in 60–70%	Borderline/moderate	Marked hypotonia, failure to thrive, delayed sexual development, scoliosis, acromicria, small stature, persistent skin picking. Typical facies: prominent forehead with bitemporal narrowing, almond-shaped eyes, triangular mouth. Up to 6 months, hypotonia, feeding difficulties and sleepiness. Later, hyperphagia arises from hypothalamic abnormalities. Psychiatric and behavioural problems increase with age.

Syndrome	Incidence	Aetiology/ genetics	Severity LD	Main features
Rett syndrome	1:10 000 females	Distal arm of Xq28 75% MECP2 mutation	Profound	Pervasive developmental disorder. Diagnostic criteria: normal development until 6–18 months, deceleration of head growth, loss of verbal ability, stereotypic movements replace purposeful hand movements, failure to walk or abnormal gait, ataxic movements of torso/limbs worse with distress. Regression of physical, social, linguistic and adaptive behaviours. Breathing abnormalities.
Smith–Magenis syndrome	1:25 000	Partial/ complete deletion of band 17p11.2	Moderate	Multiple congenital abnormalities, hearing/visual difficulties, scoliosis, sleep disturbance. Typical facies: brachycephaly, broad face and nasal bridge, flat midface, mouth turned down, cupid's bow shaped upper lip, abnormal shape/position of ear. Self-injury, hyperactivity, aggression, need for 1:1 adult attention. Hypothyroidism, immunoglobulin deficiency, congenital heart disease.
Sturge–Weber syndrome	Uncertain; cases sporadic			Uncommon developmental disorder: unilateral/bilateral port-wine naevus (usually in distribution of trigeminal nerve), epilepsy, hemiparesis, mental impairment, eye problems (raised intraocular pressure, glaucoma/buphthalmos, field defects, choroidal naevi, colobomas of iris). Seizures focal or generalized; mostly develop in first year of life; brain damage following fits may worsen hemiplegia or mental impairment.
Tuberous sclerosis	1:7000	Autosomal dominant, 9q34.3 or 16p13.3	50% LD: severe/ profound	Complex non-degenerative, neurocutaneous multisystem condition: diverse symptoms/severity. Sclerotic tuber-like growths may affect any part of body; typically, hamartia, hamartomas neoplasia, facial angiofibromas; 50% have LD, 75% develop epilepsy, 50% show autistim-like behaviour and/or hyperactivity (irrespective of level of LD). Cerebral and renal lesions having highest mortality.

Syndrome	Incidence	Aetiology/ genetics	Severity LD	Main features
West syndrome	Depends on cause	Various congenital brain malformations	Severe	Infantile spasms—flexor (salaam) and extensor myoclonic spasms of neck, truck and links; hypsarrhythmic EEG; severe LD; onset <1 year. Common causes: Down syndrome, leucodystrophy, tuberous sclerosis, inborn errors of metabolism, prenatal infection, perinatal hypoxia.
Williams syndrome			Mild/ moderate	Progressive multisystem syndrome with elfin facies, supravalvular aortic stenosis, LD with severe visuospatial/motor deficits, hypercalcaemia. Hypercalcaemia especially in infancy. Cardiovascular features such as hypertension, arterial stenosis, mitral valve collapse. Kyphosis, scoliosis, joint contractures. Urinary and gastrointestinal problems such as constipation. Odd cognitive/ personality profile with extraordinary verbal facility.

Further reading

Aman MG, Techan CJ, White AJ, Turbott SH, Vaithiananthan C. Haloperidol treatment with chronically medicated residents. Dose effects on clinical behaviour and reinforcement contingencies. *American Journal of Mental Retardation* 1989; **93**: 452–460.

Anderson LT, Campbell M, Grega D, Perry R, Small A, Green W. Haloperidol in the treatment of infantile autism: effects on learning and behavioural symptoms. *American Journal of Psychiatry* 1984; **141**: 1195–1202.

Anderson LT, Campbell M. The effects of haloperidol on discrimination learning and behavioural symptoms in autistic children. *Journal of Autism and Developmental Disorders* 1989; **19**: 227–239.

Barak Y, Ring A, Levy D, Grande I, Szor H, Elizue A. Disabling compulsions in 11 mentally retarded adults: an open trial of clomipramine SR. *Journal of Clinical Psychiatry* 1995; **56**: 459–461.

Barrickman L, Noyes R, Kaperman S, Schumacher E, Verda M. Treatment of ADHD with fluoxetine: a preliminary trial. *Journal of the American Academy of Child and Adolescent Psychiatry* 1991; **30**: 762–776.

Bauer MS, Whybrow PC. Rapid cycling bipolar affective disorder, II. Treatment of refractory rapid cycling with high dose levothyroxine: a preliminary study. *Archives of General Psychiatry* 1990; **47**: 435–440.

Bhaumik S, Branford D, Naik BI, Biswas AB. Retrospective audit of selective serotonin re-uptake inhibitors (fluoxetine and paroxetine) of the treatment of depressive episodes in adults with learning disability. *British Journal of Developmental Disabilities* 2000; **46**: 131–139.

Birmaher B, Quintana H, Greenville L. Methyphenidate treatment of hyperactive autistic children. *Journal of the American Academy of Child and Adolescent Psychiatry* 1988; **27**: 248–251.

Bodfish JW, Madison JT. Diagnosis and fluoxetine treatment of compulsive behaviour disorder of adults with mental retardation. *American Journal of Mental Retardation* 1993; **98**: 360–367.

Branford D, Bhaumik S, Naik B. Selective serotonin reuptake inhibitors for the treatment of perseverative and maladaptive behaviours of people with intellectual disability. *Journal of Intellectual Disability Research* 1998; **42**: 301–306.

Buitelaar JR, Van der Gaag RJ, Cohen-Kettenis P, Melman CT. A randomised controlled trial of risperidone in the treatment of aggression in hospitalised adolescents with subaverage cognitive abilities. *Journal of Clinical Psychiatry* 2001; **62**: 239–248.

Calabrese JR, Bowden CL, Sachs GS, Ascher JA, Monaghan E, Rudd GD. A double blind placebo controlled study of lamotrigine monotherapy in outpatients with bipolar I depression. Lamictal 602 Study Group. *Journal of Clinical Psychiatry* 1999; **60**: 79–88.

Calabrese JR, Delnechi GA. Spectrum of efficacy of valproate in 55 patients with rapid cycling bipolar disorder. *American Journal of Psychiatry* 1990; **147**: 431–434.

Casanova M, Walker L, Whitehouse P, Price D. Abnormalities of the nucleus basalis in Down's syndrome. *Annals of Neurology* 1985; **18**: 310–313.

Cohen SA, Ihrig K, Lott RS, Kenrick JM. Risperidone for aggression and self-injurious behaviour in adults with mental retardation. *Journal of Autism and Developmental Disorders* 1998; **28**: 229–233.

Comings D, Comings B. A controlled study of Tourette syndrome 1–VII. *American Journal of Human Genetics* 1987; **41**: 701–866.

Cook EH Jr, Rowlett R, Jaselskis C, Leventhal BL. Fluoxetine treatment of children and adults with autistic disorder and mental retardation. *Journal of the American Academy of Child and Adolescent Psychiatry* 1992; **31**: 739–745.

Cooper S-A, Prasher VP. Maladaptive behaviours and symptoms of dementia in adults with Down's syndrome compared with adults with intellectual disability of other aetiologies. *Journal of Intellectual Disability Research* 1998; **42**: 293–300.

Corbett J. Psychiatric morbidity and mental retardation. In: Smith P, James FE, (eds). *Psychiatric Illness and Mental Handicap*. Ashford: Headley Brothers, 1979, pp. 11–25.

Davanzo PA, Belin TR, Widowski MH, King BH. Paroxetine treatment of aggression and self-injury in persons with mental retardation. *American Journal of Mental Retardation* 1998; **102**: 427–437.

Diagnostic and Statistical Manual of Mental Disorders, 4th edition (DSM-IV). Washington, D.C.: American Psychiatric Press, 1994.

Dommisse J. Organic mania induced by phenytoin. *Canadian Journal of Psychiatry* 1990; **35**: 457.

Dubovsky SL. Calcium channel antagonists as novel agents for manic depressive disorder. In: Schatzburg AF, Nerneroff CB (eds). *Textbook of Psychopharmacology*. Washington, DC: American Psychiatric Press, 1995, pp. 455–472.

Eames P. Traumatic brain injury. *Current Opinion in Psychiatry* 1997; **10**: 49–52.

Friedman DL, Kastner T, Plummer AT, Ruiz MQ, Henning D. Adverse behaviour effects in individuals with mental retardation and mood disorder treated with carbamazepine. *American Journal of Mental Retardation* 1992; **96**: 541–546.

Forsgren I, Edvinsson SO, Blomquist HK, Heijbel J, Sidenvall R. Epilepsy in a population of mentally retarded children and adults. *Epilepsy Research* 1990; **6**: 234–248.

Gillberg C, Persson U, Grufman M, Temner U. Psychiatric disorders in mildly and severely mentally retarded urban children and adolescents: epidemiological aspects. *British Journal of Psychiatry* 1986; **149**: 68–74.

Goate A, Chartier-Harlan M, Mullan M et al. Segregation of a mis-sense mutation in the amyloid precursor protein gene with familial Alzheimer's disease. *Nature* 1991; **349**: 704–706.

Goodman R, Stevenson J. A twin study of hyperactivity. I. An examination of hyperactivity scores and categories derived from Rutter Teacher and Parent questionnaires. II. The aetiological role of genes, family relationships and perinatal adversity. *Journal of Child Psychology and Psychiatry* 1989; **30**: 671–710.

Gordon C, Rapoport J, Hamburger S, State R, Mannheim G. Differential response of seven subjects with autistic disorder to clomipramine and desipramine. *American Journal of Psychiatry* 1992; **149**: 363–366.

Gordon CT. Commentary: consideration of the pharmacological treatment of compulsions and stereotypes with serotonin reuptake inhibitors in pervasive developmental disorders. *Journal of Autism and Developmental Disorders* 2000; **30**: 437–438.

Griffin JC, Ricketts RW, Williams DE, Locke BJ, Altmeyer BK, Stark MT. A community survey of self-injurious behaviour among developmentally disabled children and adolescents. *Hospital and Community Psychiatry* 1987; **38**: 959–963.

Handen BL, Johnson CR, Lubetsky M. Efficacy of methyphenidate among children with autism and symptoms of attention deficit hyperactivity disorder. *Journal of Autism and Developmental Disorders* 2000; **30**: 245–255.

Happe F. Parts and wholes, meaning and minds: central coherence and its relation to theory of mind. In: Baron-Cohen S, Tager-Flusberg H, Cohen DJ (eds). *Understanding Other Minds*, 2nd edition. Oxford: Oxford University Press, 2000, pp. 222–252.

Hauser W, Annegers J, Karland L. Incidence of epilepsy in unprovoked seizures in Rochester, Minnesota 1935–1984. *Epilepsia* 1993; **34**: 453–468.

Heaton-Ward WA. Psychosis in mental handicap. *British Journal of Psychiatry* 1977; **130**: 524–533.

Henriksen O, Bjomaes H, Roste AK. Epilepsy surgery in mental retardation; the role of surgery. In: Sillanpaa M, Gram L, Johannessen SI, Tomson T (eds). *Epilepsy and Mental Retardation*. Philadelphia: Wrightson Biomedical, 1999, pp. 105–113.

Horrigan JP, Barnhill LJ. Risperidone and explosive aggression in autism. *Journal of Autism and Developmental Disorders* 1997; **27**: 313–323.

Howland R. Fluoxetine treatment of depression in mentally retarded adults. *Journal of Nervous and Mental Disease* 1992; **180**: 202–205.

International Statistical Classification of Diseases and Related Health Problems, 10th revision (ICD-10). Geneva: World Health Organisation, 1992.

Jablensky, A. Epidemiology of schizophrenia: a European perspective. *Schizophrenia Bulletin* 1986; **12**: 52–73.

Jaleskis C, Cook EH Jr, Fletcher R, Leventhal B. Clonidine treatment of hyperactive and impulsive children with autistic disorder. *Journal of Clinical Psychopharmacology* 1992; **12**: 322–327.

Jan JE, Espezel H. Melatonin treatment of chronic sleep disorder. *Developmental Medicine and Child Neurology* 1995; **37**: 279–280.

Jenkins R, Lewis G, Bebbington P et al. The National Psychiatric Morbidity Surveys of Great Britain—initial findings from the household survey. *Psychological Medicine* 1997; **27**: 775–789.

Jervis GA. Early senile dementia mongoloid idiocy. *American Journal of Psychiatry* 1948; **105**: 102–106.

Kemner C, Van Engelend H, Tuynman-Qua H. An open-label study of olanzapine in children with PDD. *Schizophrenia Research* 2000, **41**: 194.

Koeppen D, Baruzzi A, Capozza M et al. Clobazam in therapy-resistant patients with partial epilepsy: a double-blind placebo-controlled cross-over study. *Epilepsia* 1987; **28**: 495–506.

Kubacki A. Sexual disinhibition on clonazepam. *Canadian Journal of Psychiatry* 1987; **32**: 643–645.

Maj M, Pirozzi R, Magliano L, Baroli L. Long-term outcome of lithium prophylaxis in bipolar disorder: a 5-year prospective study of 402 patients at a lithium clinic. *American Journal of Psychiatry* 1998; **155**: 30–35.

Mann DMA, Esirin MM. The pattern of acquisition of plaques and tangles in the brains of patients under 50 years of age with Down syndrome. *Journal of the Neurological Sciences* 1989; **89**: 169–179.

Masi G, Marchesci M, Pfanner P. Paroxetine in depressed adolescents with intellectual disability—an open label study. *Journal of Intellectual Disability Research* 1997; **41**: 268–272.

Maudsley Prescribing Guidelines, 7th edition. Bethlem and Maudsley NHS Trust. London: Martin Dunitz, 2003.

McDonough M, Hillary J, Kennedy N. Olanzapine for chronic stereotypic self-injurious behaviour: a pilot study in seven adults with intellectual disabilities. *Journal of Intellectual Disabilities Research* 2000; **44**: 677–684.

McDougle CJ, Holmes JP, Carlson DC, Petton GH, Cohen DJ, Price LH. A double-blind, placebo-controlled study of risperidone in adults with autistic disorders and other pervasive developmental disorders. *Archive of General Psychiatry* 1998; **55**: 633–641.

McDougle CJ, Kresch LE, Posey OJ. Repetitive thoughts and behaviour in pervasive developmental disorders: treatment with serotonin reuptake inhibitors. *Journal of Autistic and Developmental Disorders* 2000; **30**: 427–435.

McGrother CW, Hauck A, Bhaumik S, Thorp CF, Taub N. Community care for adults with learning disability and their carers: needs and outcome from the Leicestershire Register. *Journal of Intellectual Disability Research* 1996; **40**: 183–190.

Mikati MA, Choueri R, Khurana DS, Riviello J, Helmers S, Holmes G. Gabapentin in the treatment of refractory partial epilepsy in children with intellectual disability. *Journal of Intellectual Disability Research* 1998; **42** (Suppl 1): 57–62.

Moss S, Patel P. Dementia in older people with intellectual disability: symptoms of physical and mental illness and levels of adaptive behaviour. *Journal of Intellectual Disability Research* 1997; **41**: 60–69.

Perry R, Campbell M, Adams P et al. Long-term efficacy of haloperidol in autistic children: continuous versus discontinuous drug administration. *Journal of the American Academy of Child and Adolescent Psychiatry* 1989; **28**: 87–92.

Posey DJ, Litwiller M, Kohburn A, McDougle CJ. Paroxetine in autism. *Journal of the American Academy of Child and Adolescent Psychiatry* 1999; **38**: 111–112.

Potenza MN, Holmes JP, Kanes SJ, McDougle CJ. Olanzapine treatment of children, adolescents and adults with pervasive developmental disorders: an open-label pilot study. *Journal of Clinical Psychopharmacology* 1999; **19**: 37–44.

Prasher VP, Corbett JA. Onset of seizure as a poor indicator of longevity in people with Down syndrome and dementia. *International Journal of Geriatric Psychiatry* 1993; **8**: 923–927.

Ratey J, Bemporad J, Sorgi P et al. Brief report: open trial effects of beta-blockers on speech and social behaviours in 8 autistic adults. *Journal of Autism and Developmental Disorders* 1987; **17**: 439–446.

Ratey J, Sovner R, Parks A, Rogantine K. Buspirone treatment of aggression and anxiety in mentally retarded patients. A multiple-baseline, placebo lead-in study. *Journal of Clinical Psychiatry* 1991; **52**: 159–162.

Reid AH. Psychosis in adult mental defectives. *British Journal of Psychiatry* 1972; **120**: 205–218.

Ricketts RW, Goza AB, Ellis CR et al. Clinical effects of buspirone on intractable self-injury in adults with mental retardation. *Journal of American Academy of Child Adolescent Psychiatry* 1994; **33**: 270–276.

Rinh HA, Crellin R, Kirker S, Reynolds H. Vigabatrin and depression. *Journal of Neurology, Neurosurgery and Psychiatry* 1993; **56**: 925–928.

Rojahn J. Self-injurious and stereotypic behaviour of non-institutionalised mentally retarded people. Prevalence and classification. *American Journal of Mental Deficiency* 1986; **91**: 268–276.

Rojahn J. Epidemiology and topographic taxonomy of self-injurious behaviour. In: Thompson T, Gray DB (eds). *Destructive Behaviour in Developmental Disabilities*. London: Sage Publications, 1994, pp. 49–67.

Ruedrich SL, Grush L, Wilson J. Beta adrenergic blocking medications for aggressive or self-injurious mentally retarded persons. *American Journal of Mental Retardation* 1990; **95**: 110–119.

Rumble B, Retallack R, Hilbich C, Simms G, Mulhaup G, Martins R. Amyloid A4 protein and its precursors in Down's syndrome and Alzheimer's disease. *New England Journal of Medicine* 1989; **320**: 1446–1452.

Sajatovic M, Ramirez LF, Kenny JT, Meltzer HY. The use of clozapine in borderline intellectual functioning and mentally retarded schizophrenic patients. *Comprehensive Psychiatry* 1994; **35**: 29–33.

Sandman CA, Baron JL, Chicz-DeMet A, DeMet EM. Plasma β endorphin levels in people with self-injurious behaviour and stereotypy. *American Journal of Mental Retardation* 1990; **95**: 84–92.

Shaywitz B, Cohen DR, Bower M. CSF monoamine metabolites in children with minimal brain dysfunction: evidence of alteration of brain dopamine. A preliminary report. *Journal of Paediatrics* 1977; **90**: 671–677.

Sinet PM. Metabolism of oxygen derivatives in Down syndrome. *Annals of the New York Academy of Sciences* 1982; **396**: 83–94.

Strayhorn J, Rapp N, Donina W, Strain P. Randomised trial of methyphenidate for an autistic child. *Journal of the American Academy of Child and Adolescent Psychiatry* 1998; **27**: 244–247.

Struss D, Benson D. Cognition and memory. In: Perecman E (ed). *The Frontal Lobes Revisited*. New York: IRBN Press, 1984.

Todd RD. Fluoxetine in autism (Letter). *American Journal of Psychiatry* 1991; **148**: 1089.

Tohen M, Sanger TM, McElroy SL and the Olanzapine HGEH Group. Olanzapine versus placebo in the treatment of acute mania. *American Journal of Psychiatry* 1999; **156**: 702–709.

Tsiouris JA, Patti PJ. Drug treatment of depression associated with dementia or presented as 'pseudodementia' in older adults with Down syndrome. *Journal of Applied Research in Intellectual Disability* 1997; **10**: 312–322.

Tusk J, Hill P. Behavioural phenotypes in dysmorphic syndromes. *Clinical Dysmorphology* 1995; **4**: 105–115.

Vanden BR, Vermote R, Pattiens M, Thiry P. Risperidone as add-on therapy in behavioural disturbances in mental retardation. A double blind placebo-controlled cross-over study. *Acta Psychiatrica Scandinavica*, 1993; **87**: 167–170.

Victoroff J, Benson D, Grafton S, Engel J Jr, Mazziotta JC. Depression in complex partial seizures: electroencephalography and cerebral metabolic correlates. *Archives of Neurology* 1994; **51**: 155–163.

Williams CA, Tiefenbach S, McReynolds JW. Valproic acid-induced hyperammonaemia in mentally retarded adults. *Neurology* 1984; **34**: 550–553.

Wisniewski H, Rabe A. Discrepancy between Alzheimer-type neuropathology and dementia in persons with Down syndrome. *Annals of the New York Academy of Sciences* 1986; **477**: 247–260.

Wright EC. The presentation of mental illness in mentally retarded adults. *British Journal of Psychiatry* 1982; **141**: 496–502.

Zigman W, Silverman W, Winiewski HM. Ageing and Alzheimer's disease in Down syndrome: clinical and pathological changes. *Mental Retardation and Developmental Disability Research Review* 1996; **2**: 1–7.

Index